Managing Sciatica
and Radicular Pain
in Primary Care Practice

W0051314

Development of this book was supported by funding from Pfizer

Managing Sciatica and Radicular Pain in Primary Care Practice

Editors
Dr Françoise Laroche
Saint-Antoine University Hospital,
Paris, France;
President, Circle of Pain Studies in Rheumatology

Professor Serge Perrot
Hôtel-Dieu Hospital Pain Clinic,
Paris, France;
Vice President, Circle of Pain Studies in Rheumatology

Contributors
Joanne L. Jordan, Systematic Reviewer
Kika Konstantinou, Spinal Physiotherapy Specialist
Paolo Marchettini, Pain Pathophysiology and Therapy Specialist
Ana Navarro-Siguero, General Practitioner
Maria Teresa Saldaña, General Practitioner
Noelia Sánchez, Pain Unit Nurse
Concepción Pérez Hernández, Chronic and Interventional Pain Specialist
Kees Vos, Primary Care Physician
Brad Williamson, Consultant in Spinal Surgery

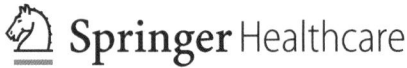

Springer Healthcare

Published by Springer Healthcare Ltd, 236 Gray's Inn Road, London, WC1X 8HB, UK.

www.springerhealthcare.com

© 2013 Springer Healthcare, a part of Springer Science+Business Media.

British Library Cataloguing-in-Publication Data.

A catalogue record for this book is available from the British Library.

ISBN 978-1-907673-55-9

Although every effort has been made to ensure that drug doses and other information are
presented accurately in this publication, the ultimate responsibility rests with the prescribing
physician. Neither the publisher nor the authors can be held responsible for errors or for any
consequences arising from the use of the information contained herein. Any product mentioned
in this publication should be used in accordance with the prescribing information prepared by
the manufacturers. No claims or endorsements are made for any drug or compound at present
under clinical investigation.

Project editor: Tamsin Curtis
Designer: Joe Harvey
Artworker: Sissan Mollerfors
Production: Marina Maher
Printed in Great Britain by Latimer Trend

Contents

Author biographies

Editors

Dr Françoise Laroche is a rheumatologist in the Pain Evaluation and Treatment Department of Saint-Antoine University Hospital in Paris, France. Dr Laroche is President of the French Pain Studies in Rheumatology Circle (CEDR), the French group of rheumatologists involved in the pain field, which is a section of the French Rheumatology Society (SFR). She has an MA in Clinical Pharmacology and is expert in chronic pain treatment and in cognitive-behavioural therapy (CBT). She implements and organises the rheumatology, pain management and CBT for chronic pain education at the University of Paris since 1993, and she is responsible for the University Diploma for Chronic Pain Management with CBT. Dr Laroche is also Clinical Researcher at the INSERM Unit (Physiopathology and Clinical Pharmacology of Pain) at the Paré Hospital, Boulogne, since 2007 and is a Medical Expert in pain and rheumatology at the French Drug Agency, since 1998. She is a member of several societies, including International Association for the Study of Pain (IASP) and the French Pain Society (SFETD).

Professor Serge Perrot is a rheumatologist with a special interest in pain management. He is currently Head of the Hôtel-Dieu Hospital Pain Clinic, Paris, France. Professor Perrot is the founder and current Vice President of CEDR, an organisation that links the SFR with the SFETD. He is in charge of coordination of teaching Pain Medicine at Paris Descartes University. He is currently providing expert guidance for the French Drug Agency on analgesics and is a member of several editorial boards for journals on pain.

Professor Perrot has participated in several workshops to establish national and international guidelines on pain management, especially on back pain. He has coordinated more than 50 studies on rheumatology in the field of pain. Professor Perrot has worked on morphine and inflammation for several years at INSERM, the French national medical research institute. His primary areas of interest are morphine and opioids in rheumatology, rheumatological pain conditions like fibromyalgia, low back pain and complex regional pain syndromes. He has developed a screening tool in fibromyalgia, the Fibromyalgia Rapid Screening Tool (FiRST). Professor Perrot is member of international scientific societies in pain and rheumatology: IASP and the European League Against Rheumatism.

Contributors

Joanne L. Jordan, is a systematic reviewer for Keele University at the Arthritis Research UK Primary Care Centre, providing support and training in aspects of systematic review methods, particularly information retrieval, giving guidance on information management, since 2004.

Ms Jordan completed a BSc in Mathematics for Business at Middlesex University and MSc in Statistics at the University of Kent in 1993, and, after completing a MA in Library and Information Science at Loughborough University, worked as an information specialist on a number of evidence-based products and publications. These include the *Clinical Effectiveness Bulletins* at Leeds University, an HTA report on chronic stable angina for Brunel University, evidence-based, shared decision-making tools for Dartmouth College in the United States, developing clinical guidelines for the Chartered Society of Physiotherapy and as an information specialist for The Cochrane Collaboration and *British Medical Journal's Clinical Evidence*.

Dr Kika Konstantinou, is a clinical academic at Keele University in the Arthritis Research UK Primary Care Centre since 2005. She has specialised in the assessment and treatment of musculoskeletal and spinal problems since 2000 and also works as a spinal physiotherapy specialist at the Haywood Hospital in Stoke-on-Trent, UK. Dr Konstantinou received a BSc in Physiotherapy, MSc in manual therapy and PhD in 2002. She leads and contributes to research programmes and projects investigating assessment and treatments for spinal and other musculoskeletal problems. Her research interests and publications are predominantly in low back pain and sciatica and in 2010 she obtained a research award for clinical epidemiological research into back pain and sciatica in primary care patients.

Professor Paolo Marchettini, is Professor of Pain Pathophysiology and Therapy at the University of the Italian Suisse canton Tessin, Switzerland and Consultant for Pain Medicine of the Department of Neurology at the Scientific Institute and Hospital San Raffaele, Italy. Dr Marchettini graduated in Medicine in 1979 at the University of Milan and then specialised in neurology and orthopaedic surgery. He trained in pain physiopathology and clinical research with Professor José Ochoa at the University of Wisconsin, USA and Professor Ulf Lindblom at the Karolinska Institute, Stockholm. From 1987 to 2005, Dr Marchettini was Director of the Pain Medicine Center of the Scientific Institute San Raffaele, Milan. His research contributions include the identification of muscle nociceptors in humans, the comparative analysis of the systemic effects of intravenous local anaesthetics in humans and rats and the clinical description of the most common iatrogenic nerve injuries. He pioneered intrathecal therapy in Italy, introducing morphine in the 1980s and recently ziconotide. Dr Marchettini serves on the editorial boards of the *European Journal of Pain*, the *Clinical Journal of Pain* and the *Pain Medicine Journal.* He is a founding member of the Gruppo Neuroscienze e Dolore (Neuroscience and Pain Group) of the Italian Neurological Society (SIN) and Member of the Swiss and Italian chapters and of IASP.

Dr Ana Navarro-Siguero is a general practitioner at the Primary Care Health Centre Puerta del Ángel in Madrid, Spain. She received a Bachelor of Medicine and Surgery degree from the Universidad Complutense de Madrid in 1992 and specialised in Family Medicine and Community MIR in 1995. Dr Navarro-Siguero was Medical Coordinator of the Health Center Angel Gate 2006–2009 and Medical Practice Teaching associate at the Department of Medicine, University Complutense of Madrid since 2009. She is a member of the Group for the Rational Use of Medicines Primary-Care Specialty Care Center District since 2011. Dr Navarro-Siguero has co-authored many articles related to pain in international journals and conference papers.

Dr Maria Teresa Saldaña is a general practitioner at the Primary Care Health Centre Raíces in Castrillón, Spain. She received her Bachelor of Medicine and Surgery from the University of Salamanca and specialised in Family and Community Medicine at the Hospital Carmen y Severo Ochoa. Dr Saldana has published many articles and reviews on acute and chronic pain.

Noelia Sánchez is a nurse in the pain unit at the University Hospital de la Princesa in Madrid, Spain. She received her Diploma in Nursing from Pontificia Comillas University. Ms Sanchez has many years of experience working in the area of pain; she has been a course instructor covering subjects such as administering medication to control pain, acute postoperative pain, pain control in nursing units, she has also tutored nursing students in clinical practice. Ms Sanchez has also been involved in the presentation of posters at pain conferences, participated as a speaker at several conferences and has been involved with more than 20 clinical trials.

Dr Concepción Pérez Hernández is Head of the Pain Clinic at the University Princess Hospital, Madrid, Spain and is responsible for Acute Postoperative Pain Unit. Dr Pérez Hernández specialises in chronic pain, particularly neuropathic pain, as well as interventional pain management.

She received her Bachelor of Medicine and Surgery at the Complutense University of Madrid and specialised in Anesthesiology, Resuscitation and Pain Therapy at the Hospital Universitario de la Princesa.

Dr Pérez Hernández is an Honorary Professor a the Universidad Rey Juan Carlos and is Honorary Professor of Surgery and Medicine at the Autonomous University of Madrid and actively participates in representative forums of pain, such as the Spanish Society of Pain (SED), Spanish Society of Anesthesiology, Reanimation and Pain, The European Society of Regional Anaesthesia & Pain Therapy and is a member of the SED and the Change Pain international and national groups.

She has participated in many clinical trials, published widely in books, monographs and articles and presented at a large number of conferences.

Dr Kees Vos is a physician at the Department of General Practice, Erasmus University, Rotterdam. He earned his MD at the Erasmus University of Rotterdam, in 1981 he completed his training in General Practice and two years later his training as a physician in Sports Medicine. In 1983, Dr Vos started as a general practitioner in Rotterdam and worked concurrently in several different facilities for Sports Medical Care and Advice. In 2002 he moved from Rotterdam and started working in a primary care centre in Spijkenisse. Between 1996 and 2004 he worked as physician at the Whiplash Centre in The Netherlands.

From the end of 1999 until 2006, Dr Vos researched acute neck pain in the Department of General Practice of the Erasmus University Rotterdam leading to his PhD thesis in 2006 and from 2001 to 2004, Dr Vos trained in Clinical Epidemiology at the EMGO Institute in Amsterdam. Since 2007 he has been the Chair of the medical advisory board of the Dutch Whiplash Patient Society. He is also a member of several national guide-line committees and advisory boards on chronic pain and is an active participant and co-author in different chronic pain research projects. He has been an active organiser and chair in continuing education courses on different medical topics and is a teacher of clinical epidemiology topics for interns.

Brad Williamson is presently Chair of Neurosciences at Salford Royal Hospital, where he has managerial responsibility for a group of 25 surgeons performing over 3000 spinal operations each year. In addition. Mr Williamson holds a number of professional affiliations, including Senior Lecturer in Healthcare Science at the University of Salford. Mr Williamson trained in Manchester and Hong Kong. In 1991, he was appointed as Senior Lecturer at the University of Manchester and Honorary Consultant in Orthopaedic Surgery. In 1995, Mr Williamson was appointed as a full time NHS consultant in spinal surgery at Hope Hospital, Salford and the Royal Manchester Children's Hospital, since then both spinal units have expanded greatly.

His practice covers all aspects of spinal disorders and he aims to provide high quality, evidence-based care for all of his patients. Mr Williamson is research active and is the author of over twenty peer-reviewed publications as well as a number of book chapters. He currently holds grants for research into the aetiology and pathogenesis of adolescent idiopathic scoliosis and wound healing in patients with spinal tumours. He has previously held the posts of President of the British Scoliosis Society, examiner for the Royal College of Surgeons (FRCS Orth) and specialist adviser to National Institute for Health and Clinical Excellence (NICE).

Development of this book was supported by funding from Pfizer

Introduction

Françoise Laroche and Serge Perrot

From pathophysiology to clinical assessment and therapeutic approaches: A single entity with specific approaches

Low back pain (LBP) is a major public health issue, with a high prevalence and constant increased burden. LBP has been cited as the second most frequent reason to visit a physician for a chronic condition, the fifth most common cause for hospitalisation and the third most frequent reason for a surgical procedure of the spinal column [1–4]. In many cases LBP is associated to sciatica and radicular pain, and studies infrequently individualise this clinical aspect, while the diagnostic and therapeutic specificities of LBP are poorly analysed and described. Numerous specialities are involved in diagnosis and management of sciatica, for example, rheumatologists, neurologists, orthopaedic surgeons, rehabilitation physicians, general practitioners, and as such there can often times be a lack of consensus on the pathophysiological concepts, assessment and treatments.

This book provides an accurate update on LBP with or without sciatica, and on related concepts and issues, such as: How can radicular pain, radiculopathy and sciatica be differentiated? Is radicular pain a neuropathic pain? What are the causes of radiculopathic pain? What are the specific risk factors for developing a radiculopathy? How can sciatica be managed?

There is an increased burden of radicular pain, with between 20% to 35% of patients with back pain suffering from a neuropathic pain component. Currently, chronic lumbar radicular pain is the most common neuropathic pain syndrome [5–10]. Not all risk factors for developing radiculopathy have been determined, but a clear correlation has been established for some factors which predispose patients to radiculopathy and back pain.

Literature on sciatica and radicular pain is frequently confusing. In this book, the authors clarify these concepts and provide clear defintions of radicular pain, radiculopathy and sciatica with supporting literature.

Mechanisms and theories

At least three mechanisms are involved in the pathophysiology of radicular pain: inflammation, immunlogical local mechanisms and local compression. The pathophysiology of radicular pain, and the specific mechanisms that may be found in different clinical conditions, like in disc herniation, diabetes, cancer, have all been summarised.

Clinical approaches

Radicular pain may be related to numerous causes. The diagnosis of a lumbosacral radiculopathy should be based on clinical examination. It is recommended that clinicians conduct a focused history and physical examination of the patient with LBP in order to classify them into the correct category of back pain, for example, nonspecific LBP, back pain possibly associated with radiculopathy or spinal stenosis, or back pain possibly associated with another specific spinal cause [11]. Several diagnostic algorithms have been provided in this book to assist clinicians with diagnosis.

Therapeutic approaches

International recommendations for the management of LBP and lumbar or cervical radiculopathy resulting from sciatica and other radicular pain syndromes are discussed in Chapter 8. All pharmacological therapies, such as nonsteroidal anti-inflammatory drugs, anticonvulsants, local steroid injections together with non-pharmacological techniques, are also discussed and put into context, including exercise, manual therapy, traction, acupuncture, passive physiotherapy interventions, electrotherapy, back braces or supports, bed rest and inactivity and psychological therapies.

In conclusion, this collaborative work will help physicians and therefore, most importantly, patients, to improve pain management, especially the undertreated and underdiagnosed radicular pain.

References

1 Anderssen GBJ. Frymoyer JW (eds). The epidemiology of spinal disorders. In: *The Adult Spine: Principles and Practice.* New York: Raven Press; 1997:93-141.

2 Cunningham LS, Kelsey JL. Epidemiology of musculoskeletal impairments and associated disability. *Am J Public Health.* 1984;74:574-579.

3 National Center for Health Statistics. Limitations of activity due to chronic conditions, United States. 1974;10:111.

4 National Center for Health Statistics. Physician visits, volume and interval since last visit, United States. 1971;10:97.

5 Baron R, Binder A. How neuropathic is sciatica? The mixed pain concept. *Orthopade.* 2004;33:568-575.

6 Freynhagen R, Baron R, Tölle TRT, et al. Screening of neuropathic pain components in patients with chronic back pain associated with nerve root compression: a prospective observational pilot study (MIPORT). *Curr Med Res Opin.* 2006;22:529-537.

7 Freynhagen R, Baron R, Gockel U, Tölle TR. painDETECT: a new screening questionnaire to identify neuropathic components in patients with back pain. *Curr Med Res Opin.* 2006;22:1911-1920.

8 Gustorff B, Dorner T, Likar R, et al. Prevalence of selfreported neuropathic pain and impact on quality of life: a prospective representative survey. *Acta Anaesthesiol Scand.* 2008; 52:132-136.

9 Hassan AE, Saleh HA, Baroudy YM, et al. Prevalence of neuropathic pain among patients suffering from chronic low back pain in Saudi Arabia. *Saudi Med J.* 2004;25:1986-1990.

10 Torrance N, Smith BH, Bennett MI, Lee AJ. The epidemiology of chronic pain of predominantly neuropathic origin. Results from a general population survey. *J Pain.* 2006;7:281-289.

11 Cowan P. Consumers' Guide Practice Guidelines For Low Back Pain. American Chronic Pain Association. 2008.

Chapter 1

What is sciatica and radicular pain?

Concepción Pérez Hernández, Noelia Sánchez,
Ana Navarro-Siguero and Maria Teresa Saldaña

One of the most frequent reasons for scheduling a primary care appointment is lumbar pain radiating to the lower leg or legs. Pain physicians often define radicular pain or sciatica as involving neuropathic mechanisms, whereas other specialists, such as rheumatologists, rehabilitation physicians and orthopaedists, do not consider neuropathy as a pathophysiological mechanism in radicular pain. This divergence in approach raises important questions about the pathophysiology of lumbar radicular pain, questions that have important assessment and therapeutic consequences.

What is sciatica and radicular pain?
How are radicular pain, radiculopathy and sciatica defined and differentiated?

To distinguish radicular pain, radiculopathy and sciatica it is important to first define a few concepts [1]. Radicular pain is defined as 'pain perceived as arising in a limb or the trunk caused by ectopic activation of nociceptive afferent fibres in a spinal nerve or its roots or other neuropathic mechanisms' [2]. It may be acute or chronic and does not necessarily entail injury to the nerve root or roots in question. It is therefore merely a pain symptom with radicular disposition.

F. Laroche and S. Perrot (eds.), *Managing Sciatica and Radicular Pain in Primary Care Practice*, DOI: 10.1007/978-1-907673-56-6_1,
© Springer Healthcare 2013

In the case of radicular pain, only radiating pain may be present, while in the case of radiculopathy, sensory and/or motor loss that can be objectified can be observed. Both syndromes frequently occur together and radiculopathy can be a continuum of radicular pain [3]. The term radiculopathy thus implies a pathological condition of a nerve root. Lumbosacral radiculopathy, like other forms of radiculopathy, results from nerve root impingement and/or inflammation that has progressed enough to cause neurological symptoms in the areas that are supplied by the affected nerve root(s). Lumbosacral radiculopathy is a condition in which a disease process affects the function of one or more lumbosacral nerve roots [4].

Finally, sciatica is a common term and one that is often used interchangeably with radicular pain and radiculopathy. Sciatica describes leg pain that is localised in the distribution of one or more lumbosacral nerve roots, typically L5-S1, with or without neurological deficit. It is equivalent to sciatic neuralgia and is defined as 'pain in the distribution of the sciatic nerve due to pathology of the nerve itself' [5]. According to these definitions, sciatic neuralgia is clearly a form of radicular pain, and is described as a disease of the peripheral nervous system. However, the term sciatica may cause confusion and physicians often use this as a label to describe leg pain from any lumbosacral segment. For this reason, some physicians have asked for this term to be removed from the medical lexicon [5]. Despite this, sciatica, when used to describe a clinical symptom (distinct from any pathophysiological considerations), is still a relevant term for patients. Most of the epidemiological and clinical studies in this area refer to pain symptoms and the focus of this chapter will be on spinal radicular pain, radiating from cervical, lumbar and, infrequently, the thoracic spine.

How is neuropathic pain defined?

Neuropathic pain is pain caused by a lesion or disease of the somatosensory nervous system. This is a clinical description that requires a demonstrable lesion or a disease that satisfies established neurological diagnostic criteria. The term 'lesion' is commonly used when diagnostic tests (eg, imaging, neurophysiology, biopsies, lab tests) reveal an abnormality or when there has been obvious trauma. The term 'disease' is commonly used when the underlying cause of the lesion is known (eg, stroke, vasculitis, diabetes mellitus, genetic abnormality). The presence of symptoms or signs (eg, touch-evoked pain) alone does not justify the use of the term 'neuropathic'. Diagnostic testing of neuropathic pain often yields inconclusive or even inconsistent data and, in such cases, clinical judgment is required to reduce all the findings in a patient into one putative diagnosis or concise group of diagnoses [6]. Several studies have investigated the neuropathic components of radicular pain, and different screening tools such as the Neuropathic Pain in 4 Questions (Douleur Neuropathique en 4 Questions; DN4) [7], painDETECT [8] and the Standardized Evaluation of Pain (StEP) [9] assessment questionnaires have yielded similar results. Using the DN4 questionnaire, Attal et al [7] concluded that neuropathic mechanisms contribute to pain both in the back area and radicular area, with the neuropathic component most pronounced in those patients with distal radiating pain in the leg.

What is the anatomy of the spinal column?

The spinal cord is located inside the vertebral canal, which is formed by the foramina of seven cervical, twelve thoracic, five lumbar and five sacral vertebrae, which together form the spine. The spinal cord extends from the foramen magnum down to the level of the first and second lumbar vertebrae (at birth, down to the second and third lumbar vertebrae).

The spinal nerves consist of the sensory nerve roots, which enter the spinal cord at each level, and the motor roots, which emerge from the cord at each level (Figure 1.1). Spinal nerve roots provide the connection between the central nervous system and the peripheral nervous system. Each nerve root is formed by the union of two roots: the motor ventral root (with the cell body, ie, soma) in the anterior horn within the cord parenchyma (see relevant reflex centre levels in Table 1.1) and the sensory dorsal root.

The cell bodies of the sensory nerves are located in the dorsal root ganglion, a key structure in the pathogenesis of radicular pain (Figures 1.2 and 1.3). Each dorsal root contains the input from all the structures within the distribution of its corresponding body segment (ie, somite). Dermatomal maps portray sensory distributions for each level, although

Spinal cord and nerves

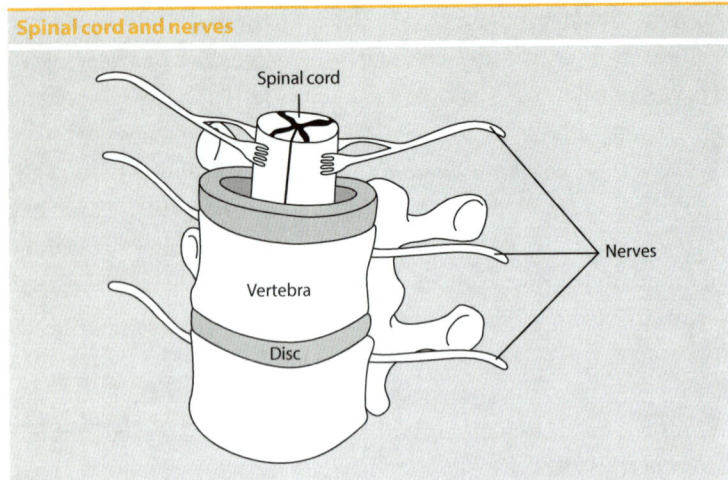

Figure 1.1 Spinal cord and nerves.

Reflex centre levels

Reflex	Level
Biceps	C5-C6
Braquioradialis	C5-C6
Triceps	C7
Finger flexors	C8
Knee	L3 (L2-L4)
Ankle	S1 (L5-S2)

Table 1.1 Reflex centre levels. The most relevant reflex and ventral root levels that are seen in clinical practice.

Spinal cord and roots

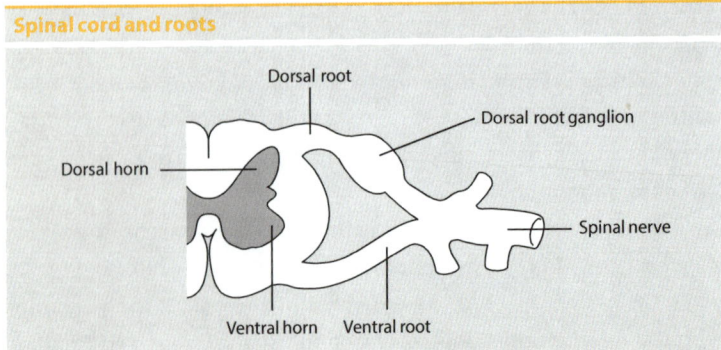

Figure 1.2 Spinal cord and roots.

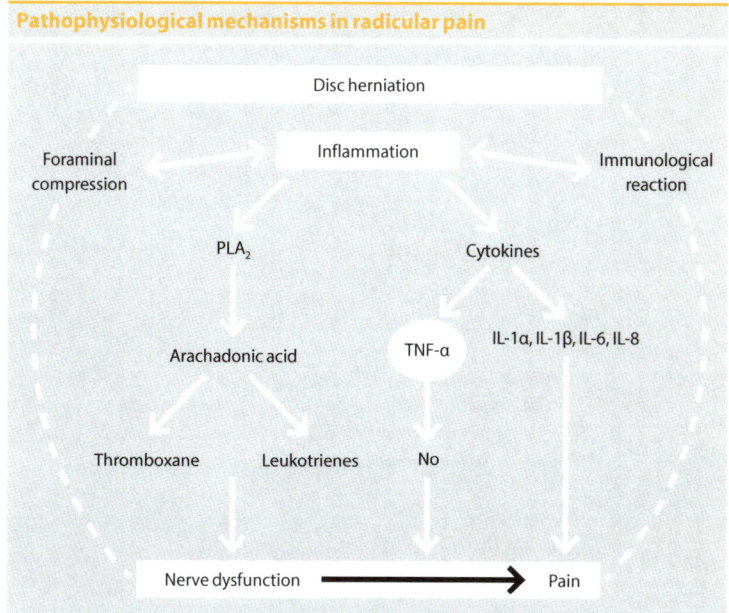

Figure 1.3 Pathophysiological mechanisms in radicular pain. Image from Stafford et al [1].
© 2007, Oxford University Press.

these maps differ somewhat according to the methods used in their construction. In addition, innervation from one dermatomal segment to another overlaps considerably (Figure 1.4, Table 1.2) [10]. The two roots come together near the dorsal root ganglion.

The external part of the spinal cord consists of white matter, while the internal part is composed of grey matter. The white matter includes the three funiculi: posterior, lateral and anterior. Each funiculus contains ascending and descending tracts. The grey matter can be divided into ten laminae/layers or into four parts: anterior or ventral horn (ie, motor neurons), posterior or dorsal horn (ie, sensory part), intermediate zones (ie, associate neurons; lamina VII) and lateral horns (where sympathetic neurons are located) [11]. It is important to emphasise that discussion of the spinal column should not be limited to the nervous system and the vertebrae. Surrounding muscles, tendons, intervertebral joints and intervertebral discs are also part of the spinal column and play an important role in pain pathophysiology.

Dermatome map of the body

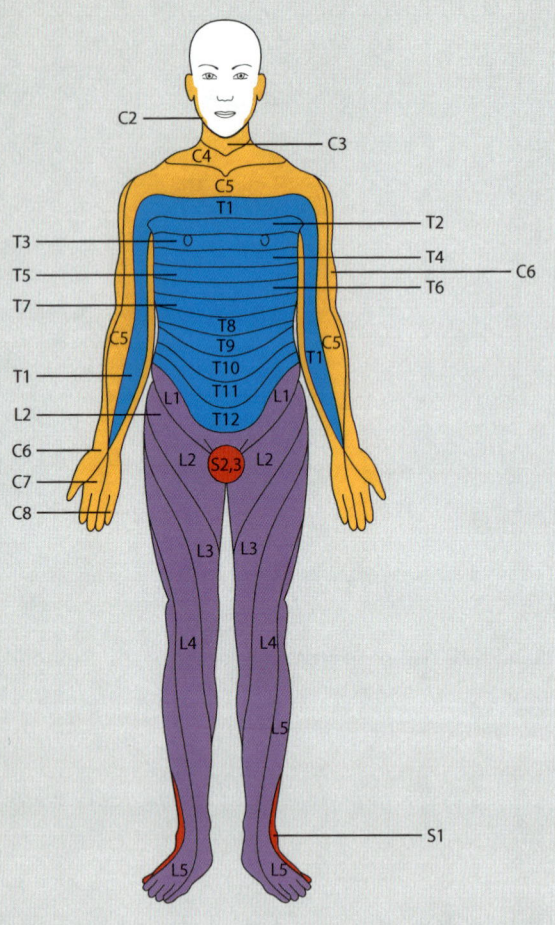

Levels of principal dermatomes

C5	Clavicles	**C8**	Ring and little fingers
C5, 6, 7	Lateral parts of upper limbs	**T3,4**	Level of nipples
C8, T1	Medial sides of upper limbs	**T10**	Level of umbilicus
C6	Thumb	**T12**	Inguinal or groin regions
C6, 7, 8	Hand	**L1, 2, 3, 4**	Anterior and inner surfaces of lower limbs

Figure 1.4 Dermatome map of the body. Reproduced with permission from Netter [10].

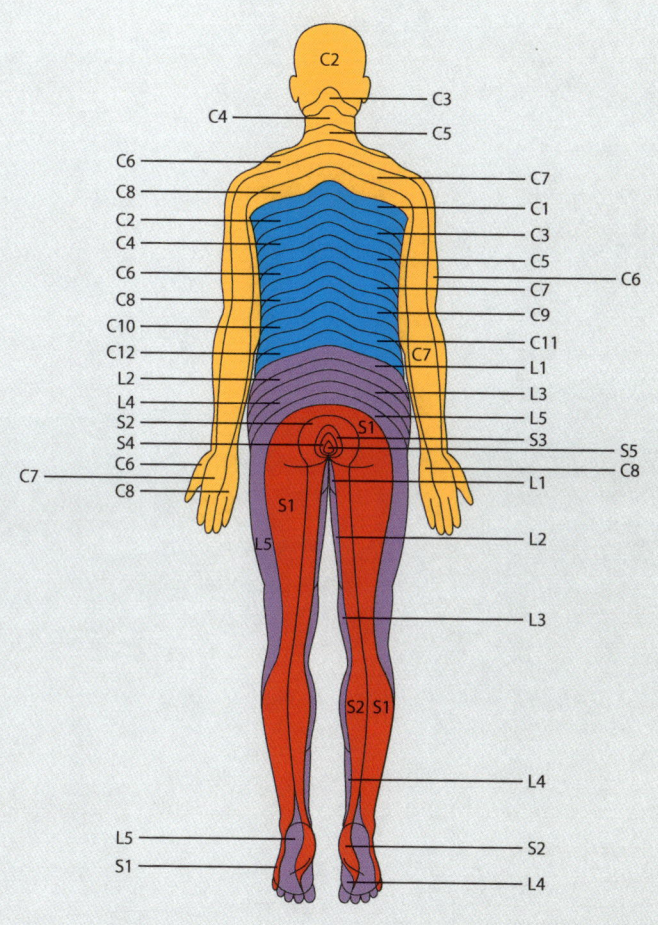

L4, 5, S1	Foot	**S1**	Lateral margin of foot and little toe
L4	Medial side of big toe		
S1, 2, L5	Posterior and outer surfaces of lower limbs	**S2, 3, 4**	Perineum

Schematic demarcation of dermatomes shown as distinct segments. There is actually considerable overlap between any two adjacent dermatomes

Dermatomal maps

Dermatomal	Cutaneous localisation
C2 and C3	Posterior head and neck
C4 and T2	Adjacent to each other in the upper thorax
T3 or T4	Nipple
T10	Umbilicus
C5	Anterior shoulder
C6	Thumb
C7	Index and middle fingers
C 7/8	Ring finger
C8	Little finger
T1	Inner forearm
T2	Upper inner arm
T2/3	Axilla
L1	Anterior upper-inner thigh
L2	Anterior upper thigh
L3	Knee
L4	Medial malleolus
L5	Dorsum of foot
L5	Toes 1–3
S1	Toes 4, 5; lateral malleolus
S3	Anus

Table 1.2 Dermatomal maps. The correlation with skin for the most clinically important dermatomes.

What is the epidemiology and incidence of spinal radicular pain?

It is difficult to determine the exact incidence of radicular pain because much of the literature in this area employs confusing terms that do not distinguish radicular from LBP, and includes both diseases that present with radicular pain or radiculopathy and diseases that do not. In addition, it is difficult to find studies that evaluate the incidence of radicular pain not just at the lumbar and sacral levels, but also at the thoracic (which is much less common) or the cervical level.

Between 80% and 90% of the general population suffers from LBP, whereas only 34–40% and 7–14% of the population suffers from cervical or thoracic spine pain, respectively [12]. Between 20% and 35% of patients with back pain suffer from radicular pain. Lumbar radicular pain is the most common neuropathic pain syndrome and its prevalence in the general population is approximately 3% to 5%, distributed equally between men and women [3,13,14], but can be much higher among certain subgroups, depending on profession. Of these cases, up to 30% last longer than one year [15,16].

The true incidence and prevalence of cervical radicular pain is uncertain; however, 51% of adults experience neck and arm pain at some time [17]. In a population-based study in Rochester, USA, the annual incidence of documented cervical radicular pain from all causes for men and women was 107.3 and 63.5 cases per 100,000 population, respectively [18]. A recent study from Europe reported a prevalence of cervical radicular pain as 1 case per 1000 people [19].

What are the risk factors for radicular pain?

The risk factors for developing radicular pain are probably different for cervical, lumbar and thoracic pain. Correlations have been described for factors that predispose patients to radicular pain, mostly lumbar radicular pain [1,4,5,20,21]:

- severe obesity (only in males in the age range of 50 to 64 years);
- age – the incidence rate peaks in the fifth decade and declines thereafter; elderly patients have an increased incidence of radiculopathies between L2 and L4;
- walking and jogging are risk factors if the patient has had previous episodes of radicular pain (if not, the activities play a protective role);
- professional activity – activity related to physical activity (eg, job function), especially flexing/twisting the trunk, frequently raising arms above shoulder height and driving motor vehicles;
- professional dancers and golf players are prone to lumbosacral radiculopathy;
- smoking;
- high serum levels of C-reactive protein.

Neither sex nor body mass have been shown to have an influence on the development of radicular pain and the role of genetic predisposition is currently unclear.

Epidemiological studies have mostly focused on back pain and it is not clear if risk factors for chronic low back (cLBP) and chronic lumbar radicular pain are different.

What is the economic burden of lumbar radicular pain?

LBP has been cited as the among the most frequent reasons to visit a physician, one of the most common causes for hospitalisation and a frequent reason for a surgical procedure [22–25]. The socioeconomic impact of cLBP is significant, although a minority of patients with cLBP and disability due to cLBP account for most of this economic burden [22]. A distinction between the burden of LBP and that of lumbar radicular pain has not been established, hence the global socioeconomic burden is generally reported for LBP, rather than for radicular pain specifically. Some estimates suggest, however, that neuropathic pain accounts for 16% of total back-pain-related costs [26].

The National Health Service in the UK spends more than £1 billion per year on costs related to back pain, which includes: £512 million on hospital costs for back pain patients, £141 million on general practitioner consultations for back pain and £150 million on physiotherapy treatments for back pain [27]. The total cost of back pain equates to between 1% and 2% of the gross national product for the UK [28]. Other European countries report similar high costs; studies have found total back-pain-related costs of €3.5 billion in The Netherlands [29] and more than €2 billion in Sweden [30].

Social and quality-of-life burden

Radicular pain includes a neuropathic element and this has important consequences in terms of the health-related quality of life of the patient. Evidence suggests that individuals with neuropathic pain experience considerably lower health utility scores, and hence reduced health-related quality of life (HRQoL), compared with either the general population or patients with some other chronic conditions including cancer and heart failure [31]. Predictably, the more severe the neuropathic pain, the greater the reduction in health utility and HRQoL.

What are the pathophysiological mechanisms in radicular pain?

Radicular pain has both neuropathic and nociceptive components. At least three mechanisms are involved in its pathophysiology, which is probably not very different from that of common neuropathic pain [1] (Figure 1.3). One should also consider that acute and chronic pain are different, with central mechanisms being more important in chronic conditions.

Inflammatory mechanism

High levels of phospholipase A2 (PLA2), an important enzyme in the inflammatory process, have been observed in patients with radicular pain caused by disc herniation [1]. PLA2 liberates arachidonic acid, a precursor of the inflammatory mediators leukotriene B_4 and thromboxane B_2. Meanwhile, cytokines are liberated, including interleukins (IL) 1α (IL-1α), IL-1β, IL-6, IL-8, prostaglandin E2 and tumour necrosis factor-alpha (TNFα). TNFα induces the formation of nitric oxide, a potent inflammatory mediator [1].

Immunological mechanism

There is evidence to suggest an immunological mechanism may play a part in the interaction between the nerve root and the exposed nucleus pulposus. Glycosphingolipids are abundant in cells of the central and peripheral nervous system and radiculopathy has been associated with an increase in anti-GSL antibodies in patients with acute and chronic sciatica and those who had lumbar discectomy for disc herniation [32]. In addition, spinal fluid, in patients presenting for disc surgery, shows an increase in glial cell markers and nerve damage markers, such as neurofilament and S-100 protein compared with controls [33]. Immunological mechanisms seem to be active in both acute and chronic radiculopathy.

Compressive mechanism

Spinal nerve roots lack a well-developed intraneural blood–nerve barrier, and this deficiency makes them more susceptible to symptomatic compression injury. Increased vascular permeability caused by mechanical nerve-root compression can induce endoneural oedemas. Furthermore, elevated endoneural fluid pressure due to an intraneural oedema can impede capillary blood flow and cause intraneural fibrosis. In addition, spinal nerve roots receive approximately 60% of their nutrition from surrounding cerebral spinal fluid (CSF). Perineural fibrosis interferes with CSF-mediated nutrition and renders the nerve roots hyperaesthetic and sensitive to compressive forces [34].

Central mechanisms

Radicular pain does not only involve peripheral mechanisms, but also central mechanisms, especially in chronic cases [35].

What symptoms are associated with radicular pain?

The symptoms a patient with radicular pain might experience include:

- leg or arm pain, according to the condition. This pain can be persistent or the result of movement, or in some cases mainly while sitting (discogenic pain) or while walking (spinal stenosis);
- numbness and tingling in the limb;
- muscle weakness;
- neuropathic symptoms;
- LBP and loss of function and mobility.

Back pain is one of the most common problems seen by family practitioners. Lumbosacral radiculopathies produce the syndrome of sciatica; cervical radiculopathies, the syndrome of brachialgia. The root pain of sciatica is almost invariably accompanied or preceded by back pain and that of brachialgia by neck pain (therefore also referred to as cervicobrachialgia). Superimposed on a steady ache is a pain with a dull but biting quality, accompanied by excruciating spasms of the paravertebral and limb muscles. On occasion, specific areas or points along the course of the sciatic nerve are tender and painful. The dull pain associated with radiculopathy is often more prominent in the proximal supply area of the damaged nerve root. It is usually deep, referred to the muscles, bones or joints. The sharper pain is more likely to radiate along dermatomal boundaries [36] (Table 1.3).

Despite the large number of nerve roots subject to potential compromise in the lumbosacral region, approximately 80% of lumbar radiculopathies involve the L5 and S1 nerve roots (sciatica) [37]. L5 radiculopathy results in pain over the dorsum and lateral part of the foot and weakness of ankle and toe extensors and S1 radiculopathy results in overt pain in the plantar part of the foot and weakness of toe flexors [38].

Straight leg raising (SLR) with the patient lying face down that produces ipsilateral leg pain should be declared positive for disc herniation and SLR that produces pain in the opposite leg also carries a high probability of disc herniation [39–41] (see Figure 4.2). Reverse SLR may elicit symptoms of pain by irritated or compressed nerve roots (L3 and L4) in the mid-to-upper lumbar region.

Consistent myotomal weakness and sensory findings that seem to coincide with segmental radiculopathy or polyradiculopathies should not be ignored. Weakness confined to the muscles in a particular lumbosacral myotome should raise the suspicion of radiculopathy, although few patients will spontaneously report such specific complaints. Inability to get up from a chair suggests iliopsoas or quadriceps weakness, while buckling of the knee is consistent with quadriceps weakness and dragging the toe points to tibialis anterior weakness [36].

Pain and sensory symptoms such as paraesthesia, dysaesthesia, hyperaesthesia or anaesthesia that involve a specific lumbosacral dermatome are suggestive of a radicular process. Paraesthesia occurs in 63–72% of lumbosacral radiculopathy cases, radiating pain in approximately 35% of

Characteristics of pain due to nerve compression
Dermatomal distribution
May be accompanied by paraesthesia
May be accompanied by abnormal sensations such as pricking or tingling
May be accompanied by sensory loss in dermatomal distribution
Loss of power in the muscles innervated by the root

Table 1.3 Characteristics of pain due to nerve compression.

cases and numbness in approximately 27% of cases [42,43]. Differentiating the neuropathic component of back pain may be difficult in clinical practice but the painDETECT questionnaire [8] and the DN4 questionnaire for patients [7] have demonstrated utility in this area. These scales are easily administered and are therefore based exclusively on clinical descriptors and not on examination.

References

1   Stafford MA, Pang P, Hill DA. Sciatica: a review of history, epidemiology, pathogenesis, and the role of epidural steroid injection in management. *Br J Anaesth*. 2007;99:461-473.
2   Merskey H, Bogduk N. *Classification of Chronic Pain. Descriptions of Chronic Pain Syndromes and Definitions of Pain Terms*. 2nd edn. Seattle, WA: IASP Press; 1994:11-17.
3   Van Boxem K, Cheng J, Patijn J, et al. Lumbosacral radicular pain. *Pain Pract*. 2010;10:339-358.
4   Tarulli AW, Raynor EM. Lumbosacral radiculopathy. *Neurol Clin*. 2007;25:387-405.
5   Frymoyer JW. Back pain and sciatica. *N Engl J Med*. 1988;318:291-300.
6   International Association for the Study of Pain. IASP taxonomy. Available at: www.iasp-pain.org/Content/NavigationMenu/GeneralResourceLinks/PainDefinitions/default.htm. Accessed August 29, 2012.
7   Attal N, Perrot S, Fermanian J, Bouhassira D. The neuropathic components of chronic low back pain: a prospective multicenter study using the DN4 Questionnaire. *J Pain*. 2011;12:1080-1087.
8   Freynhagen R, Baron R, Gockel U, Tölle TR. painDETECT: a new screening questionnaire to identify neuropathic components in patients with back pain. *Curr Med Res Opin*. 2006;22:1911-1920.
9   Scholz J, Mannion RJ, Hord DE, et al. A novel tool for the assessment of pain: validation in low back pain. *PLoS Med*. 2009;6:e1000047.
10 Netter F. Dermatome map of the body. *Atlas of Human Anatomy*. 5th edn. Philadelphia, PA: Saunders; 2010:159.
11 Moore KL. *Clinically Oriented Anatomy*. Baltimore, MD: Williams & Wilkins; 1992.
12 Giles LGF, ed. *100 Challenging Spinal Pain Syndrome Cases*. Edinburgh, UK: Elsevier; 2009.
13 Freynhagen R, Baron R. The evaluation of neuropathic components in low back pain. *Curr Pain Headache Rep*. 2009;13:185-190.
14 Valat JP, Genevay S, Marty M, Rozenberg S, Koes B. Sciatica. *Best Pract Res Clin Rheumatol*. 2010;24:241-252.
15 Weber H, Holme I, Amlie E. The natural course of acute sciatica with nerve root symptoms in a double blind placebo-controlled trial of evaluating the effect of piroxicam (NSAID). *Spine*. 1993;18:1433-1438.
16 Vroomen PCAJ, Krom MCTFM de, Slofstra PD, Knottnerus JA. Conservative treatment of sciatica: a systematic review. *J Spinal Dis*. 2000;13:463-469.
17 Hult L. Frequency of symptoms of different age groups and professions. In: Hirsch C, Zotterman Y, eds. *Cervical Pain*. New York, NY: Pergamon Press; 1971:17-20.
18 Radhakrishnan K, Litchy WJ, O'Fallon WM, Kurland LT. Epidemiology of cervical radiculopathy. A population-based study from Rochester, Minnesota, 1976 through 1990. *Brain*. 1994;117:325-335.
19 Van Zundert J, Huntoon M, Patijn J, Lataster A, Mekhail N, van Kleef M. Cervical radicular pain. *Pain Pract*. 2010;10:1-17.
20 Kumar M, Garg G, Singh LR, Singh T, Tyagi LK. Epidemiology, pathophysiology and symptomatic treatment of sciatica: a review. *Int J Pharm Bio Arch*. 2011;2:1050-1061.
21 Shiri R, Karppinen J, Leino-Arjas P, et al. Cardiovascular and lifestyle risk factors in lumbar radicular pain or clinically defined sciatica: a systematic review. *Eur Spine J*. 2007;16:2043-2054.

22 Anderssen GBJ. Frymoyer JW (eds). The epidemiology of spinal disorders. In: The Adult Spine: Principles and Practice. New York: Raven Press; 1997:93-141.

23 Cunningham LS, Kelsey JL. Epidemiology of musculoskeletal impairments and associated disability. Am J Public Health. 1984;74:574-579.

24 National Center for Health Statistics. Limitations of activity due to chronic conditions, United States. 1974;10:111.

25 National Center for Health Statistics. Physician visits, volume and interval since last visit, United States. 1971;10:97.

26 Schmidt CO, Schweikert B, Wenig CM, et al. Modelling the prevalence and cost of back pain with neuropathic components in the general population. Eur J Pain. 2009;13:1030-1035.

27 Maniadakis A, Gray A. The economic burden of back pain in the UK. Pain. 2000;84:95-103.

28 Norlund AI, Waddell G. Cost of back pain in some OECD countries. In: Nachemson AL, Jonsson E, eds. Neck and Back Pain: The Scientific Evidence of Causes, Diagnosis and Treatment. Philadelphia, PA: Lippencott: Williams & Wilkins; 2000:421-425.

29 Lambeek LC, van Tulder MW, Swinkels ICS, et al. The trend in total cost of back pain in the Netherlands in the period 2002 to 2007. Spine. 2011;36:1050-1058.

30 Van Tulder M. Chapter 1: Introduction. Eur Spine J. 2006;15:S134-S135.

31 Doth AH, Hansson PT, Jensen MP, Taylor RS. The burden of neuropathic pain: a systematic review and meta-analysis of health utilities. Pain. 2010;149:338-344.

32 Brisby H, Balague F, Schafer D, et al. Glycosphingolipid antibodies in serum in patients with sciatica. Spine. 2002;27:380-386.

33 Brisby H, Olmarker K, Rosengren L, Cederlund CG, Rydevik B. Markers of nerve tissue injury in the cerebrospinal fluid in patients with lumbar disc herniation and sciatica. Spine. 1999;24:742-746.

34 Wheeler AH. Low back pain and sciatica. Available at: emedicine.medscape.com/article/1144130-overview. Accessed August 29, 2012.

35 Tinazzi M, Fiaschi A, Rosso T, Faccioli F, Grosslercher J, Aglioti SM. Neuroplastic changes related to pain occur at multiple levels of the human somatosensory system: a somatosensory-evoked potentials study in patients with cervical radicular pain. J Neurosci. 2000;20:9277-9283.

36 Chou R, Qaseem A, Snow V, et al; for the Clinical Efficacy Assessment Subcommittee of the American College of Physicians and the American College of Physicians/American Pain Society Low Back Pain Guidelines Panel. Diagnosis and treatment of low back pain: a Joint Clinical Practice Guideline from the American College of Physicians and the American Pain Society. Ann Intern Med. 2007;147:478-491.

37 Dumitru D, Amato AA, Zwarts M, et al. Electrodiagnostic Medicine. 2nd edn. Philadelphia, PA: Hanley and Belfus Inc.; 2002.

38 Lee-Robinson A, Lee AT. Clinical and diagnostic findings in patients with lumbar radiculopathy and polyneuropathy. Am J Clin Med. 2010;7:80-86.

39 Devillé WL, van der Windt DA, Dzaferagić A, Bezemer PD, Bouter LM. The test of Lasègue: systematic review of the accuracy in diagnosing herniated discs. Spine. 2000;25:1140-1147.

40 Rubinstein SM, van Tulder M. A best-evidence review of diagnostic procedures for neck and low-back pain. Best Pract Res Clin Rheumatol. 2008;22:471-482.

41 van der Windt DA, Simons E, Riphagen II, et al. Physical examination for lumbar radiculopathy due to disc herniation in patients with low-back pain. Cochrane Database Syst Rev. 2010;17:CD007431.

42 Norlen, G. On The Value of Neurological Symptoms in Sciatica for Localization of a Lumbar Disc Herniation. Stockholm, Sweden: P. A. Norstedt & Söner; 1944.

43 Brown HA, Pont ME. Disease of lumbar discs. Ten years of surgical treatment. J Neurosurg. 1963;20:410-417.

Development of this book was supported by funding from Pfizer

Chapter 2

What are the causes of sciatica and radicular pain?

Concepción Pérez Hernández, Noelia Sánchez,
Ana Navarro-Siguero and Maria Teresa Saldaña

Radicular pain may arise from a number of causes, including neoplastic, infectious and inflammatory disorders (Table 2.1). The diagnosis of a lumbosacral radiculopathy is clinical and can usually be made based upon compatible symptoms and examination findings. Elucidation of triggering and alleviating factors may also be helpful. Radicular pain that worsens following the Valsalva manoeuvre or improves while lying down suggests a compressive origin. Conversely, radicular pain that worsens with lying down suggests an inflammatory or neoplastic origin. However, such symptoms have not been shown to be sensitive or specific for these conditions. Bowel/bladder symptoms, particularly new urinary incontinence, suggest cauda equina syndrome [1,2].

Disc herniation and foraminal stenosis due to spondylotic degeneration are the most common aetiologies for lumbosacral radiculopathy and clinical symptoms are self-limiting in most cases. Thus, immediate diagnostic testing is not necessary for patients with suspected radiculopathy who are neurologically intact, except when there are signs that alert the clinician to a need for an exhaustive aetiological diagnosis, such as signs pointing to a neoplastic, infectious or inflammatory origin. Depending on the suspected cause, we may choose imaging, laboratory or electrophysiological studies as our complementary tests. Computed

F. Laroche and S. Perrot (eds.), *Managing Sciatica and Radicular Pain in Primary Care Practice*, DOI: 10.1007/978-1-907673-56-6_2, © Springer Healthcare 2013

Causes of lumbosacral radiculopathy

Skeletal causes	Neoplasic causes	Nonskeletal causes
Intervertebral disc herniation	Primary tumours	Diabetes mellitus
Spinal stenosis	Ependymoma	Diabetic amyotrophy
Spondylosis	Schwannoma	Single or multiple radiculopathies
Spondylolisthesis	Neurofibroma	Inflammatory disorders
Trauma	Lymphoma	Acute inflammatory demyelinating polyradiculoneuropathy (Guillain-Barré syndrome)
Piriformis syndrome	Lipoma	Arachnoiditis
	Dermoid	Chronic inflammatory demyelinating polyradiculoneuropathy
	Epidermoid	Sarcoidosis
	Haemangioblastoma	Paget's disease
	Paraganglioma	Infectious diseases
	Ganglioneuroma	Borrelia burgdorferi (Lyme disease)
	Osteoma	Cytomegalovirus
	Plasmacytoma	Epstein-Barr
	Metastatic tumours	Herpes simplex virus
	Leptomeningeal metastasis	Human immunodeficiency virus (HIV)
	Lymphoma	Mycobacterium
	Multiple myeloma	Mycoplasma
	Metastasis	Spinal epidural abscess
		Syphilis
		Varicella zoster virus (herpes zoster or shingles)
		Vascular
		Arteriovenous malformation
		Radiation-induced vascular occlusion
		Vasculitis (nerve root infarction)

Table 2.1 Causes of lumbosacral radiculopathy. Skeletal causes are common. Neoplasic causes are less frequent, with the most common being metastasis and multiple myeloma. The rest of these are rare or extremely rare (metastasis are the same as metastasic tumour). In the nonskeletal causes, diabetes, Guillain-Barré syndrome, polyradiculoneuropathy and infectious diseases are uncommon. The rest are rare or extremely rare.

tomography (CT) and magnetic resonance imaging (MRI) are the most specific imaging modalities [3].

Among all the other electrodiagnostic methods (nerve conduction examination, late responses, somatosensory evoked potentials, root electrical and magnetic stimulation examinations), the needle electrode (needle electromyography [EMG]) examination may be useful but is not a specific or sensitive diagnostic tool. In many cases, EMG may be normal, even in painful situations. In some cases, it may be helpful to differentiate radiculopathy from neuropathy. A good grasp of the anatomical, clinical and electromyographic myotomal charts is essential to localise radiculopathies to single (or more) root lesions. It is important to note that this will not provide data during the initial phase (the first 3 weeks) and it may be normal in patients with pure sensory radiculopathy, EMG should not be performed in common sciatica or lumbar radiculopathy. It should be restricted to difficult diagnostic cases or when neurologic damage assessment is mandatory.

The need for diagnostic tests becomes particularly apparent if so-called diagnostic or prognostic 'red flags' are present at any time, which may indicate an increased risk of serious pathology (Table 2.2). Diagnostic tests are also necessary in low-risk patients (those without red flags) who do not respond properly to treatment or who are candidates for more invasive therapies. Initial complementary testing is particularly important in cases of suspected neoplasia, suspected epidural abscess, radiculopathy with rapidly progressive neurological deficits and radiculopathy

Diagnostic red flags

- Pain unrelieved by rest or any postural modification
- Severe morning stiffness as the primary complaint
- Patients unable to ambulate or care for self
- Pain unchanged despite treatment for 2–4 weeks
- Writhing pain behaviour
- Colicky pain or pain associated with a visceral function
- Known or previous cancer
- Fever or immunosuppressed status
- Associated malaise, fatigue or weight loss
- High risk for fracture (eg, older age, osteoporosis)
- Progressive neurological impairment
- Bowel or bladder dysfunction

Table 2.2 Diagnostic red flags.

Yellow flags
• Dissociation between verbal and nonverbal pain behaviours
• Compensable cause of injury
• Nonorganic signs and symptoms
• Out of work, disabled or seeking disability
• Narcotic or psychoactive drug requests
• Psychological features, including depression and anxiety
• Repeated failed surgical or medical treatment for low back pain or other chronic illnesses

Table 2.3 Yellow flags.

with urinary retention and saddle anaesthesia (to rule out cauda equina compression) [4].

'Yellow flags' are psychosocial indicators suggesting increased risk of progression to long-term distress, disability and pain and they were designed for use in diagnosing acute low back pain [5,6]. Yellow flags can relate to the patient's attitudes and beliefs, emotions, behaviours, family and workplace; it is worth noting that the behaviour of health professionals can also have a major influence [7]. Identifying yellow flags may help when improvement in low back pain is delayed and the presence of yellow flags may highlight the need to address specific psychosocial factors as part of a multimodal management approach (Table 2.3) [5–7].

Skeletal causes of radiculopathy

The major causes of sciatica are compression, from disc herniation, and degenerative causes (spondyloarthropathies) that lead to spondylolisthesis and spinal stenosis (normally lumbar), which are increasingly commonplace with increasing age.

Lumbar bulging or herniated disc

Intervertebral disc herniation is the most common cause of lumbosacral radiculopathy in patients under 50 years of age. Beginning at approximately 30 years of age, the intervertebral discs undergo degenerative changes, such as dehydration and the loss of volume and elasticity, causing the disc to become less resistant. The annulus fibrosus, which covers the nucleus pulposus and acts as a shock absorber for blows and strain, may lose its stabilising properties, allowing the nucleus to shift posteriorly (disc

Lumbar bulging or herniated disc

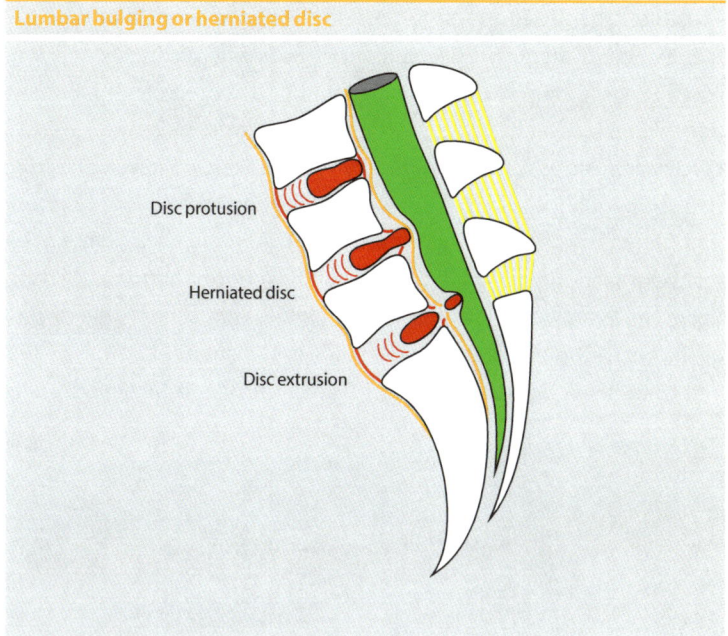

Disc protusion

Herniated disc

Disc extrusion

Figure 2.1 Lumbar bulging or herniated disc.

protrusion). The annulus fibrosis may even break, causing the nucleus to shift even more. Disc herniation (Figure 2.1) is most frequent in the cervical (C5-C6-C7) and lumbar/sacral spine (L4-L5-S1) as these areas of the spine are the most mobile [8].

A bulging disc is also known as a contained disc disorder. This means the gel-like centre (nucleus pulpous) remains enclosed within the tire-like outer wall (annulus fibrosus) of the disc. A herniated disc occurs when the nucleus breaks through the annulus. It is called a non-contained disc disorder. The disc material contains inflammatory mediators (eg, phospholipase A2, cytokines and prostaglandins) that causes nerve inflammation. In both cases, nerve compression and irritation cause inflammation and pain, often leading to extremity numbness, tingling and muscle weakness. The straight leg raising test (also called Lasegue's sign) is specific to disc herniation and can be performed bilaterally in important and median disc herniations.

Lumbar spinal stenosis

Lumbar spinal stenosis is a common, often asymptomatic, entity, that can be caused by a variety of congenital or acquired conditions. The most common origin is degenerative spondylosis. In general we can define stenosis as a nerve compression disorder most often affecting mature people. With advancing age, intervertebral discs desiccate and flatten, transferring increasing axial load to the facet joints, with resultant facet joint hypertrophy, osteophyte formation and thickening of the ligamentum flavum. These changes contribute to narrowing of the central spinal canal, lateral recesses and neural foramina. L4-5 and L5-S1 levels in particular are affected. Chronic radiculopathy may

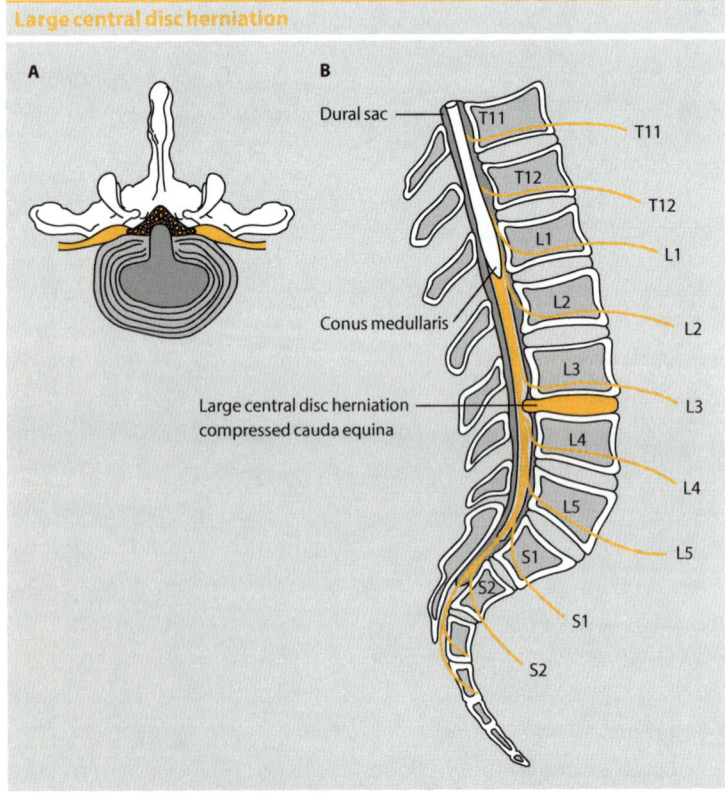

Figure 2.2 Large central disc herniation. A, Axial view. B, Sagittal view of lumbar spine.

result from entrapment of nerve roots in the lateral recess, intervertebral foramen or central canal and can involve single or multiple nerve roots. Clinical syndromes of radicular pain involving buttock, hip or posterior thigh and intermittent neurogenic claudication are more common than back pain [3].

The major manifestation of lumbar spinal stenosis is neurogenic claudication, a syndrome of bilateral, often asymmetric, pain, sensory loss and/or weakness affecting the legs. The symptoms are produced or exacerbated by walking or prolonged standing in an erect posture. In a few patients with lumbar spinal stenosis, fixed nerve root injury may occur, causing lumbosacral radiculopathy and, rarely, cauda equina syndrome or conus medullaris syndrome. Cauda equina syndrome (Figure 2.2) is caused by an intraspinal lesion caudal to the conus that injures two or more of the 18 nerve roots that constitute the cauda equina

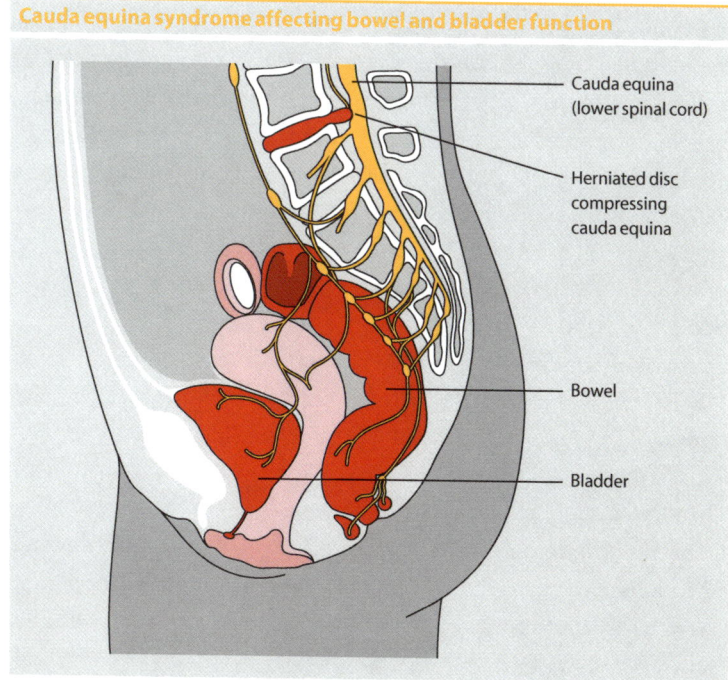

Cauda equina syndrome affecting bowel and bladder function

Cauda equina (lower spinal cord)

Herniated disc compressing cauda equina

Bowel

Bladder

Figure 2.3 Cauda equina syndrome affecting bowel and bladder function.

within the lumbar spinal canal. The clinical presentation is dominated by bilateral leg weakness in multiple root distributions (L3-S1) and may be associated with perineal sensory symptoms as well as bowel, bladder and sexual dysfunction due to involvement of the S2-4 spinal nerve roots (Figure 2.3).

Spondylosis and spondylolisthesis
Spondylosis
This is a term with many definitions and it has been used in the literature in many different contexts and employed synonymously with arthrosis, spondylitis, hypertrophic arthritis and osteoarthritis. In other instances, spondylosis is considered mechanistically as the hypertrophic response of vertebral bone adjacent to disc degeneration (although osteophytes may infrequently form in the absence of diseased discs). Finally, spondylosis may be applied nonspecifically to any and all degenerative conditions affecting the discs, vertebral bodies and/or associated joints of the lumbar spine. This is a broad definition of spondylosis, recognising the high incidence of coincident degenerative changes, and the dynamic interplay between adjacent discs, vertebra and nerves that create the clinical pain syndromes within the axial spine and associated nerves. These conditions cause pain by placing pressure on spinal nerves, resulting in symptoms such as radicular pain.

Spondylolisthesis
Spondylolisthesis is a disorder that most often affects the lumbar spine. In a normal spine the vertebrae are stacked one on top of the other, separated by discs, to form a single column. In spondylolisthesis one vertebra slips forward and off the vertebra below it, disturbing spine alignment. This slip may be slight or severe; in the worst cases of spondylolisthesis, the affected vertebra slips completely off of its support, resulting in a condition called spondyloptosis. When a vertebra slips and is displaced, spinal nerve root compression occurs and often causes radicular leg pain. It is categorised as developmental (found at birth, develops during childhood) or acquired from spinal degeneration, trauma or physical stress (ie, weightlifting).

Similarities between spondylosis and spondylolisthesis

Spondylosis is an umbrella term used to describe age-related degenera-tion of the spine. Spondylolisthesis is a specific condition in which a vertebra slips off the supporting vertebra below it. While spondylosis is a fairly common condition in people over 40 years of age, by comparison spondylolisthesis is a rare spinal defect. Although spondylolisthesis can occur at any age, degenerative spondylolisthesis is most common in people over the age of 65 years, with women having a greater risk than men.

Although they are two very different conditions with different causes, spondylosis and spondylolisthesis present in similar ways: back pain and stiffness, possible tingling and numbness in the back and legs, gradual worsening of symptoms, and potential for a loss of bladder or bowel control. Treatment plans are also similar for both conditions [9].

Trauma

Radicular pain can result from direct nerve compression caused by external forces to the lumbar or sacral spinal nerve roots, such as those arising from motor vehicle accidents, falls and sports. The impact may injure the nerves or occasionally fragments of broken bone may compress the nerves.

Piriformis syndrome

Piriformis syndrome is named after the piriformis muscle and the pain caused when the muscle irritates the sciatic nerve. The piriformis muscle is located in the lower part of the spine and connects to the thigh bone, assisting in hip rotation. The position of the sciatic nerve relative to the piriformis muscle is subject to anatomical variation and, in some indi-viduals, passes through rather than around the muscle (Figure 2.4). Contraction of the piriformis muscle may then lead to compression and inflammation of the sciatic nerve, with resultant neuralgia. Piriformis syndrome occurs most frequently in adults aged 30–40 years [10], in women more often than men and in keen sportsmen and -women. Estimates suggest that piriformis syndrome accounts for at least 6% of patients diagnosed with LBP [10–12] and nearly 70% of those with sci-atica [13]. This condition can be treated with an injection of steroid to reduce inflammation or botulinum toxin to the muscle to reduce tone [14].

Nonskeletal causes of radiculopathy

Infectious diseases

Cytomegalovirus

Cytomegalovirus radiculitis occurs in immunosuppressed patients with very low CD4 counts. It is characterised by severe paraesthesia, sensory

Anatomical variations in the relationship of the sciatic nerve to the piriformis muscle

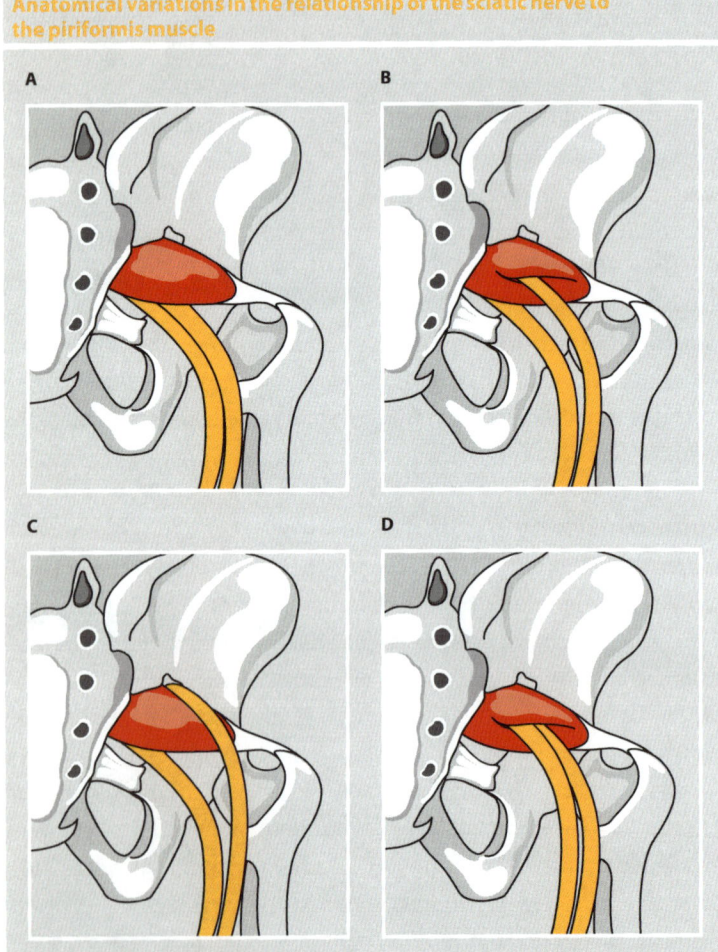

A

B

C

D

Figure 2.4 Anatomical variations in the relationship of the sciatic nerve to the piriformis muscle. A, Normal sciatic nerve and piriformis muscle; B, Sciatic nerve passes through the muscle; C, Sciatic nerve passes directly over the top the muscle; D, Sciatic nerve passes through the muscle.

loss and weakness. Both small and large nerve fibres are involved. There may also be bowel and bladder dysfunction from diminished sphincter tone [15].

Herpes zoster

Primary infection with the varicella zoster virus leads to chickenpox, usually in children, after which herpes zoster colonises the dorsal root ganglion. The virus may remain latent for years but can be reactivated decades later, producing acute herpes zoster or shingles. Reactivation is associated with a haemorrhagic lymphocytic infiltration of the ventral roots. This is a common disorder which is particularly prevalent in immunocompromised and elderly populations.

Patients present with an erythematous vesicular maculopapular rash in the dermatome of the affected root that lasts for 3–5 days. Sensory changes characterised by marked allodynia often follow. The pain of acute herpes zoster, frequently overwhelming at the outset, gradually subsides as the vesicles crust over in most patients. Approximately 10% to 15% of patients suffer from chronic pain, or postherpetic neuralgia, despite treatment with antiviral agents for herpes zoster. Herpes zoster usually affects a single dermatome; lumbosacral zoster accounts for approximately 20% of cases. Approximately 5% of patients may develop local neuritis of the spinal nerve, which subsequently affects the motor axons, producing a segmental zoster paresis. Complete resolution of motor deficits occurs in 50% to 70% of these patients [16,17].

Individual vaccines against varicella zoster and against herpes zoster are now available in some parts of the world. The varicella zoster vaccine is recommended for all children under 13 years and for older individuals who have never had chickenpox. The herpes zoster vaccine is recommended for adults over 50 years old who are most at risk of shingles.

Other infections

Other infectious causes of radicular pain are rare but they should be considered in differential diagnoses. They include *Borrelia burgdorferi*, Epstein-Barr virus, *Mycobacterium*, *Mycoplasma*, syphilis and epidural abscess.

Diabetic amyotrophy or diabetic proximal neuropathy

Diabetic amyotrophy is an uncommon diabetic neuropathy with a specific clinical profile and treatment that presents in the limbs and affects nerve roots or proximal nerves. Root infarction may occur from either large or small vessel disease. Diabetic amyotrophy is more common in diabetics with microvascular affectation. The most characteristic signs of diabetic amyotrophy are sudden-onset weakness in the pelvic-femoral area, including the L2, L3 and L4 nerve roots, in patients older than 50 years of age with type 2 diabetes, loss of deep tendon reflexes, dysaesthesia and intense pain. Significant weight loss is present in 50% of cases and its pathophysiology is primarily immunological [18,19].

Mass lesion or malignancy

Spinal tumours are abnormal growths that are either benign or cancerous (malignant). Fortunately, spinal tumours are rare. However, when a spinal tumour develops there is a risk of developing radiculopathy as a result of nerve compression.

Generally speaking, radiculopathy may develop due to tumours in various locations within the spinal canal; these lesions are usually extramedullary. Primary tumours tend to be intradural, whereas metastatic lesions are extradural. Furthermore, primary lesions tend to be solitary (neurofibromatosis type 1 being a notable exception), whereas multiple metastatic lesions frequently occur [1–3,20].

Primary nerve root tumours are a rare cause of lumbosacral radiculopathy. Most primary spinal tumours are benign and slow growing and their clinical manifestations may be difficult to distinguish from more common causes of radiculopathy, such as disc herniation. Both are characterised by back pain; however, the nature of pain related to tumour is distinctive, as it becomes increasingly severe over time and is worse when lying down, often interfering with sleep. Any new presentation with pain in a nerve root distribution, or change in a previously stable pain state, should be carefully investigated to exclude infective or malignant causes of pain. Primary tumours producing lumbosacral radiculopathy most frequently are neurofibromas (often associated with neurofibromatosis type 1) and ependymomas; less common are schwannomas (in neurofibromatosis type 2), meningiomas, lipomas and dermoids. Ependymomas and neurofibromas typically affect the filum terminale, producing a cauda equina syndrome. Diagnosis of primary tumours is established by MRI.

Epidural and vertebral metastases

Although metastatic tumour is the most common type of neoplasm involving the spinal canal, it is rare in the general population. Approximately 30% of epidural metastases occur in the lumbar spine and radicular pain is an initial symptom in approximately half of these cases [21,22]. Metastases typically invade the spinal column and extend from there into the epidural space. Metastases seed the vertebrae by way of Batson's venous plexus, which connects the deep pelvic veins and thoracic veins (draining the interior organs such as the bladder) to the internal vertebral venous plexuses. Less commonly, paravertebral lesions spread directly to nerve roots through the intervertebral neural foramina [23].

The three most common cancer metastases involving the lumbosacral spine are breast, lung and prostate cancer, each accounting for approximately 10% to 20% of cases [23].

Leptomeningeal metastases/meningeal carcinomatosis

Cancer cells may infiltrate the leptomeninges and subarachnoid space diffusely, leading to a syndrome reflecting involvement of cranial nerves, spinal nerve roots and the brain. Manifestations include radiculopathy, cranial polyneuropathy, headache, memory loss, seizures and gait disturbances. Radicular discomfort is the most common presenting symptom, usually involving lumbosacral levels resulting from involvement of the cauda equina [24]. Although all cancers have the potential to produce this condition, the most likely primary tumours to do so are leukaemia, lymphoma and breast carcinoma. Other tumours that may produce leptomeningeal metastases include melanoma, lung cancer, gastrointestinal cancers and sarcoma [25].

Other nonskeletal causes of radiculopathy

Inflammatory causes

A differential diagnosis must be performed to rule out causes of acute inflammatory demyelinating polyradiculoneuropathy (eg, Guillain-Barré syndrome), chronic inflammatory demyelinating polyradiculoneuropathy, arachnoiditis related to post-surgical changes, chemical radiculitis and the presence of sarcoidosis. Inflammatory causes are infrequent, with the exception of arachnoiditis from postsurgical changes, which is not unusual.

Vascular causes

Vascular causes of radiculopathy are rare and include arteriovenous malformation, vasculitis (with nerve root infarction) and radiation-induced vascular occlusion [26].

References

1   Giles LGF, ed. *100 Challenging Spinal Pain Syndrome Cases*. Edinburgh, UK: Elsevier; 2009.
2   McMahon S, Koltzenburg M, eds. Root disorders and arachnoiditis. In: *Wall and Melzack´s Textbook of Pain*. Philadelphia, PA: Elsevier/Churchill-Livingstone; 2005:1056-1069.
3   Tarulli AW, Raynor EM. Lumbosacral radiculopathy. *Neurol Clin*. 2007;25:387-405.
4   Kulcu DG, Naderi S. Differential diagnosis of intraspinal and extraspinal non-discogenic sciatica. *J Clin Neurosci*. 2008;15:1246-1252.
5   New Zealand Guidelines Group. New Zealand Acute Low Back Pain Guide: The Guide to Assessing Psychosocial Yellow Flags in Acute Low Back Pain (2005). Available at: www.acc.co.nz/PRD_EXT_CSMP/groups/external_communications/documents/guide/prd_ctrb112930.pdf. Last accessed December 10, 2012.
6   Kinkade S. Evaluation and treatment of acute low back pain. Am Fam Physician. 2007;75:1181-1188, 1190-1192.
7   Hunter New England Local Health District. Pain matters: red and yellow flags. Medical Practice Guidelines, NSW Government. Updated Nov 2005. Available at: www.hnehealth.nsw.gov.au/__data/assets/pdf_file/0003/28164/Guideline_flags.pdf. Last accessed December 10, 2012.
8   Frymoyer JW, Moskowitz RW. Spinal degeneration. Pathogenesis and medical management. In: Frymoyer JW, ed. *The Adult Spine: Principles and Practice*. New York, NY: Raven; 1991:611-634.
9   Middleton K, Fish DE. Lumbar spondylosis: clinical presentation and treatment approaches. *Curr Rev Musculoskelet Med*. 2009;2:94-104.
10 Papadopoulos EC. Piriformis syndrome and low back pain: a new classification and review of the literature. *Orthop Clin North Am*. 2004;35:65-71.
11 Pace JB, Nagle D. Piriformis syndrome. *West J Med*. 1976;124:435-439.
12 Hallin RP. Sciatic pain and the piriformis muscle. *Postgrad Med*. 1983;74:69-72.
13 Filler AG, Haynes J, Jordan SE, et al. Sciatica of nondisc origin and piriformis syndrome: diagnosis by magnetic resonance neurography and interventional magnetic resonance imaging with outcome study of resulting treatment. *J Neurosurg: Spine* 2005;2:99-115.

14 Benzon HT, Katz JA, Benzon HA, Iqbal MS. Piriformis syndrome: anatomic considerations, a new injection technique and a review of the literature. *Anaesthesiol*. 2003;98:1422-1428.

15 Anders HJ, Goebel FD. Cytomegalovirus polyradiculopathy in patients with AIDS. *Clin Infect Dis*. 1998;27:345-352.

16 Chad, DA. Disorders of nerve roots and plexuses. In: Bradley WG, Daroff RB, Fenichel GM, et al, eds. *Neurology in Clinical Practice*. 4th edn. Philadelphia, PA: Elsevier; 2004:2267.

17 Braverman DL, Ku A, Nagler W. Herpes zoster polyradiculopathy. *Arch Phys Med Rehabil*. 1997;78:880-882.

18 Vinik AI, Strotmeyer ES, Nakave AA, Patel CV. Diabetic neuropathy in older adults. *Clin Geriatr Med*. 2008;24:407-435.

19 Dyck PJB, Windebank AJ. Diabetic and non-diabetic lumbosacral radiculoplexus neuropathies: new insights into pathophysiology and treatment. *Muscle Nerve*. 2002;25:477-491.

20 Freeman TB, Cahill DW. Tumours of the meninges, cauda equina, and spinal nerves. In: Menezes AH, Sonntag VKH, eds. *Principles of Spinal Surgery*. New York, NY: McGraw-Hill; 1996:1371-1386.

21 Schiff D, O'Neill BP, Suman VJ. Spinal epidural metastasis as the initial manifestation of malignancy: clinical features and diagnostic approach. *Neurology*. 1997;49:452-456.

22 Helweg-Larsen S, Sorensen PS. Symptoms and signs in metastatic cord compression: a study of progression from first symptom until diagnosis in 153 patients. *Eur J Cancer*. 1994;30A:396-398.

23 Schiff D. Spinal cord compression. *Neurol Clin North Am*. 2003;21:67-86.

24 Posner JB. *Neurologic Complications of Cancer*. Philadelphia, PA: F.A. Davis Company; 1995.

25 Viali S, Hutchinson DO, Hawkins TE, et al. Presentation of intravascular lymphomatosis as lumbosacral polyradiculopathy. *Muscle Nerve*. 2000;23:1295-1300.

26 Benny BV, Nagpal AS, Singh P, Smuck M. Vascular causes of radiculopathy: a literature review. *Spine J*. 2011;11:73-85.

Development of this book was supported by funding from Pfizer

Chapter 3

How are sciatica and spinal radicular pain classified?

Ana Navarro-Siguero, Concepción Pérez Hernández and
María Teresa Saldaña

Radicular pain may be classified according to its duration and anatomical location. Most practitioners [1] classify back pain according to the length of time it persists:

- acute: lasting less than 6 weeks;
- subacute: from 7 to 12 weeks;
- chronic: more than 3 months.

What are the classifications by region of the spine?

Radicular pain is classified as cervical, thoracic or lumbar, depending on the anatomical location of the affected nerve root (see Figure 3.1).

The cervical spine is formed by seven vertebrae. Spinal nerves are named and numbered according to the point at which they emerge from the spinal canal. Nerves C1-C7 each emerge above their respective vertebrae in the cervical region and C8 emerges between the seventh cervical vertebra and the first thoracic vertebra. The cervical plexus (roots C1-C4) innervates the anterior and posterior musculature of the neck and transmits sensitivity in the skin of the face, neck and shoulders. The brachial plexus (roots C5-C8 and T1) innervates the shoulder muscles, the lower scalenes and the muscles and skin of the upper limbs. The thoracic spine is made up of twelve vertebrae and twelve nerve roots.

F. Laroche and S. Perrot (eds.), *Managing Sciatica and Radicular Pain in Primary Care Practice*, DOI: 10.1007/978-1-907673-56-6_3, © Springer Healthcare 2013

Each thoracic nerve emerges below its corresponding vertebra. The lumbar spine is formed by five vertebrae and five nerve roots that are numbered according to the vertebra immediately above it. Therefore, nerve root L1 emerges from the L1-L2 space, and the last, L5, emerges between L5 and S1 (Figure 3.1).

Because the spinal cord is not the same length as the vertebral column, cervical nerve roots run horizontally to reach the intervertebral foramen, while thoracic and lumbar nerve roots descend obliquely. Finally, the sacral and coccygeal nerve roots form the cauda equina.

Neck pain, cervical pain and cervical radiculopathy

The International Association for the Study of Pain (IASP) defines cervical spinal pain as pain perceived anywhere in the posterior region of the cervical spine, from the superior nuchal line to the first dorsal vertebra [2,3]. This definition does not include pain in the anterior part of the neck.

The Bone and Joint Decade 2000–2010 Task Force on Neck Pain and Its Associated Disorders describes neck pain as that which is located in the anatomical region of the neck with or without radiation to the head, trunk and upper limbs [4]. This definition draws the boundaries of the posterior region of the neck from the superior nuchal line to the spine of the scapula, and laterally from the superior border of the clavicle and the suprasternal notch. The Task Force's definition is more extensive than that of the IASP as it delimits the areas for the pain in question.

Cervical radiculopathy (cervicobrachialgia) is caused by the compression and inflammation of a cervical nerve. The most common causes, which may be isolated or combined, are cervical spondyloarthritis and disc herniation. Although cervical osteoarthritis is very common, most patients do not experience radicular pain. Rather, they feel somatic pain in the affected ligaments and deep joints. Bogduk and McGuirk [5] indicate that it is difficult to distinguish between this type of somatic pain and radicular pain in some cases, but that radicular pain is associated with neurological signs and is generally accompanied by paraesthesia, tingling, loss of strength and/or loss of deep tendon reflexes. Cervical radiculopathy manifests as neck pain that radiates to the upper arm and may or may not be accompanied by loss of strength and/or paraesthesia.

Anatomy of the spinal column

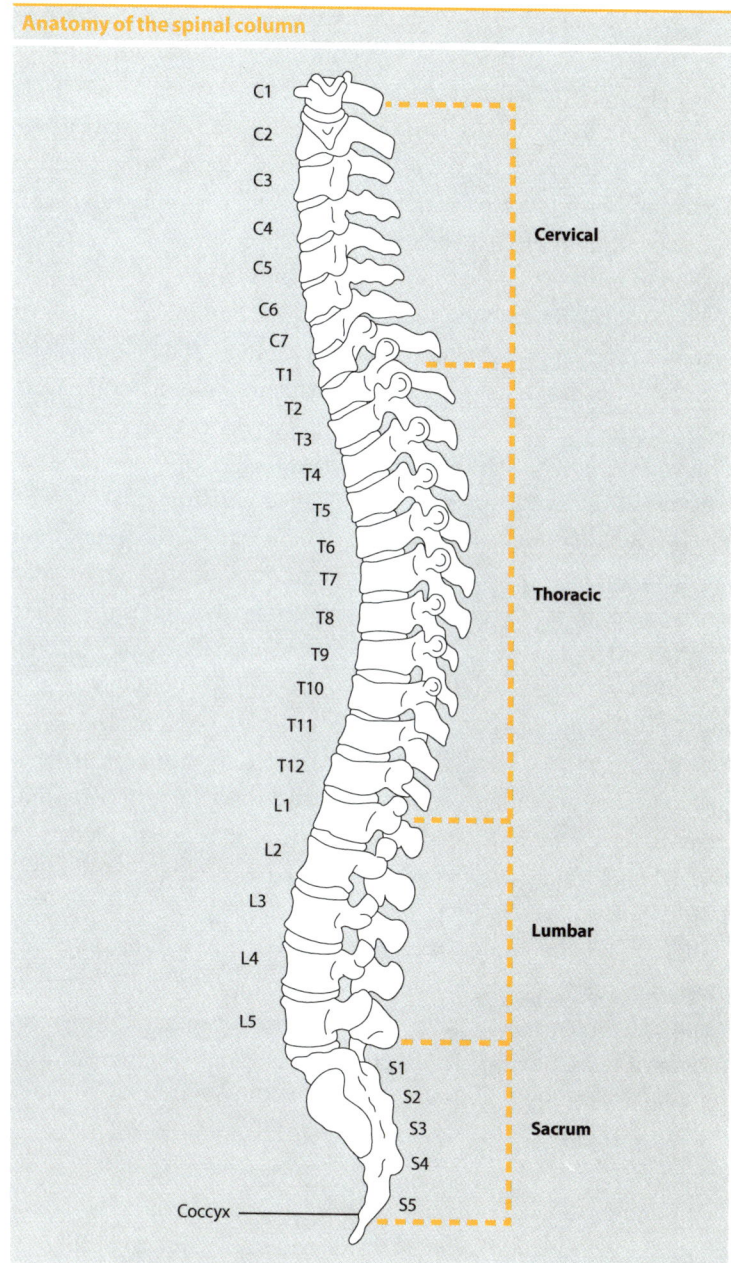

Figure 3.1 Anatomy of the spinal column.

Irritation of the cervical root produces continuous pain with neuropathic characteristics (eg, paraesthesia, dysaesthesia), which worsens with neck and arm movement and does not improve with rest, making sleep difficult. Examination often finds decreased neck mobility and muscle contraction.

C5 radiculopathy causes pain in the neck, shoulder and medial border of the scapula accompanied by paraesthesia in the lateral part of the upper arm (over the deltoids) as well as weakness in the shoulder abduction (first 90° of elevation supraspinatus, second 90° abduction deltoids), shoulder external rotation (infraspinatus muscle), shoulder internal rotation (subscapularis and teres minor) and elbow flexion (biceps). C6 radiculopathy is the most common type of cervical radiculopathy, which causes pain and/or paraesthesia in the lateral area of the arm and forearm and the thumb and index finger. Patients experience weakness in elbow supination, forearm pronation, wrist extension and pincer movement. and affects the brachioradial reflex. The second most common type is C7 radiculopathy, which causes pain and/or paraesthesia in the posterior area of the arm and forearm and the middle finger and affects the tricipital reflex. It causes weakness in elbow extension and wrist flexion (C7-C8). Radiculopathy C8 causes weakness in finger flexion and finger extension (C7-C8). In T1 radiculopathy patients feel weakness in thumb abduction and in C8-T1 radiculopathy, weakness in finger abduction and adduction. Figures 3.2 and 3.3 show the typical explorations for the most common types of cervical and lumbar radiculopathies and Tables 3.1 and 3.2 show the positive and negative signs from such investigations, respectively [6–8].

In the absence of a 'gold standard' diagnostic tool, the diagnosis of cervical radiculopathy is based on a combination of history, clinical examination and (potentially) complementary examination. Medical imaging may show abnormalities but these findings may not correlate with the patient's pain [9].

Certain physical examination manoeuvres can help in diagnosing cervical radiculopathy:

- Spurling's test: as the doctor stands behind the patient and exerts downward pressure on the head, the patient tilts his/her head to the side where the pain is, bringing the ear towards the shoulder.

This tends to trigger or accentuate pain by reducing the intervertebral foramina.
- Cervical traction test: relieves symptoms.
- Valsalva manoeuvre: worsens herniated disc pain due to increased intraspinal pressure.
- Homolateral upper limb tension test (with the doctor's hand on the patient's head) tends to lessen pain.
- Brachial plexus stretch test: with the arm on the affected side abducted to 90°, the patient hyperextends that arm with posterior and inferior traction, with the head flexed laterally towards the opposite side. This manoeuvre tends to worsen or trigger pain.

In 2007, Rubinstein et al performed a systematic review of provocative neck tests used to diagnose cervical radiculopathy [10]. They concluded that provocative tests performed on individuals with suspected cervical radiculopathy helped establish the diagnosis, particularly in subjects lacking well-defined neurological deficits. When consistent with the clinical history and other physical findings, a positive Spurling test, traction/neck distraction test and Valsalva manoeuvre might be suggestive of cervical radiculopathy, while a negative upper limb tension test might be used to rule it out. With the lack of clinical data, the values from the tests must be interpreted cautiously. Cervical radiculopathy must be distinguished from compressive cervical myelopathy and is considered a key component in the diagnostic process. The presence of pyramidal signs such as hyperreflexia, Hoffmann reflex, clonus and Babinski sign is a hallmark of myelopathy [11].

These signs, if present, can be elicited by deep tendon reflex testing with a reflex hammer. To elicit the Hoffman response, the physician holds the patient's middle finger and asks them to completely relax their fingers. The physician then presses their thumbnail down on the patient's fingernail and moves it down and along the nail until it 'clicks' over the end. An immediate brief flick of the other fingers indicates a positive Hoffman response and the presence of an upper motor neuron lesion in that arm. To test the Babinski, or plantar, reflex the physician presses the end of the reflex hammer on the side of the heel and runs

Cervical radiculopathy exploration

C5	C6

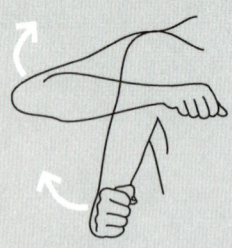

Shoulder abduction
First 90° of elevation – supraspinatus
Second 90° of elevation – deltoid

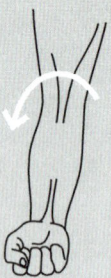

Elbow supination
Supinator

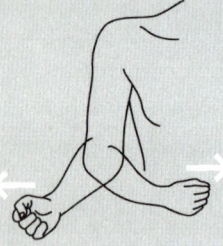

Shoulder external rotation
Infraspinatus

Shoulder internal rotation
Subscapularis, teres minor

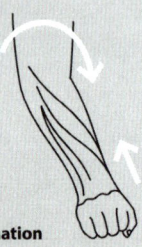

Forearm pronation
Pronator teres
Pronator quadratus (C8, T1)

Wrist extension
Extensor carpi (i) radialis longus,
(ii) radialis brevis and (iii) ulnaris

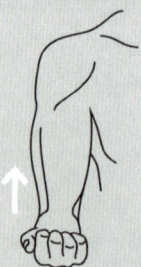

C5–6
Elbow flexion
Biceps

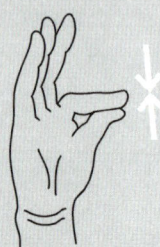

Pincing movement
Long flexor of thumb
Long flexor of index

Figure 3.2 Cervical radiculopathy exploration. Image adapted from Giles [6]. © 2009, Elsevier.

C7	C8

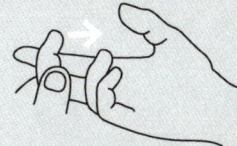

Finger flexion
Flexor digitorum (i) profundus and
(ii) superficialis

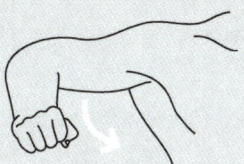

Shoulder abduction
Flexor digitorum (i) profundus and
(ii) superficialis

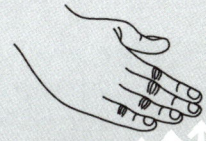

C7–8
Finger extension
Extensor (i) digitorum communis,
(ii) digiti indicis and (iii) digiti minimi

T1

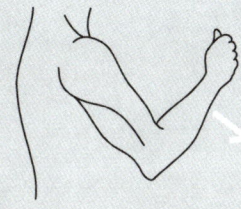

Elbow extension
Triceps

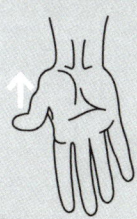

Thumb abduction
Abductor pollicis brevis

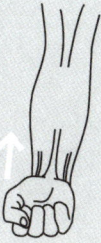

C7–8
Wrist flexion
Flexor carpi (i) radialis and (ii) ulnaris

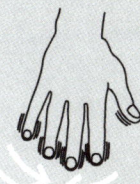

C8–T1
Finger abduction and adduction
Dorsal interossei and abductor digiti minimi

Cervical radiculopathy explorations

Cervical nerve root (disc level)	Pain	Motor weaknesses	Reflexes tested	Exam	Findings (response)
C5 (C4–C5)	Lateral arm to upper elbow, medial scapula	Deltoid, supraspinatus, infraspinatus, rhomboids	Subscapalaris, teres minor, biceps	Shoulder abduction, shoulder external and internal rotation	*Shoulder abduction:* **Normal to fair:** completes range of motion to 90° with maximal to no resistance **Poor:** palpable or visible contraction of deltoid with no movement **None:** no contractile activity *Shoulder external rotation:* **Normal to fair:** completes range of motion with maximal to no resistance **Poor:** completes available range of motion while in prone position **Trace:** contractile activity but no motion **None:** no palpable or visible activity *Shoulder internal rotation:* **Normal to fair:** completes range of motion with maximal to no resistance **Poor:** completes available range of motion **Trace:** palpable contraction **None:** no palpable contraction

| C6 (C5-C6) | Lateral forearm to thumb and index finger | Wrist extensors, biceps, forearm pronators and supinators, brachioradialis | Long flexor of thumb and finger, extensor carpi radialis longus, radialis brevis and ulnaris | Elbow flexion, wrist extension, forearm pronation and supination | *Elbow flexion:*
Normal to fair: completes range of motion with maximal to no resistance
Poor: completes partial range of motion in each muscle tested
Trace: palpable contractile response
None: no palpable contractile activity

Wrist extension:
Normal to fair: completes full range of motion with maximal to no resistance (when testing all three extensor muscles)
Poor: completes full range of motion without assistance of gravity
Trace: any muscle may exhibit visible or palpable contractile activity, but there is no wrist motion
None: no contractile activity

Forearm pronation:
Normal to fair: completes available range of motion with maximal to no resistance
Poor: completes partial range of motion
Trace: visible or contractile activity with no motion
None: no contractile activity

Forearm supination:
Normal to fair: completes full range of motion with maximal to no resistance
Poor: completes partial range of motion
Trace: slight contractile activity but no limb movement
None: no contractile activity |

Table 3.1 Cervical radiculopathy explorations (continues overleaf).

Cervical radiculopathy explorations (continued)

Cervical nerve root (disc level)	Pain	Motor weaknesses	Reflexes tested	Exam	Findings (response)
C7 (C6–C7)	Triceps, front and back of mid-forearm to middle finger, medial border of scapula	Triceps, wrist extensors and flexors, pectoralis major, latissimus dorsi, pronator teres	Triceps, flexor carpi radialis and ulnaris	Shoulder adduction, elbow extension, wrist flexion, finger extension	*Shoulder adduction:* **Normal to fair:** completes range of motion with maximal to no resistance **Poor:** palpable contractile activity **None:** no contractile activity *Elbow extension:* **Normal to fair:** completes range of motion with maximal to no resistance **Poor:** completes available range of motion without assistance of gravity **Trace:** there is tension in the triceps tendon just proximal to the olecranon or contractile activity in the muscle fibres on the arm's posterior surface **None:** no evidence of muscle action *Wrist flexion:* **Normal to fair:** completes range of motion with maximal to no resistance **Poor:** completes available range of flexion without assistance of gravity **Trace:** one or both tendons may exhibit visible or palpable contractile activity, but they do not move **None:** no contractile activity *Finger extension:* **Normal to fair:** completes active range of motion with maximal to no resistance **Poor:** completes range of motion **Trace:** visible tendon activity but no joint motion **None:** no contractile activity

| C8 (C7-T1) | Neck to shoulder, medial forearm to ring and little finger | Thumb and finger flexors, hand intrinsic muscles, abductors | Flexor digitorum profundus and superficialis, extensor digitorum communis, digiti indicis and digiti minimi | Finger flexion, thumb and forefinger pinching | *Finger flexion:*
Normal to fair: completes range of motion with maximal to no resistance
Poor: completes full range of motion
Trace: palpable visible or contractile activity
None: no contractile activity |
| T1 (T1-T2) | Shoulder and axilla to olecranon | Small muscles in hand | Dorsal interossei and abductor digiti minimi, abductor pollicis brevis | Finger abduction and adduction, thumb abduction | *Finger abduction:*
Normal or good: little resistance in the dorsal interossei and abductor digiti minimi
Fair: can abduct any given finger
Poor: completes partial range of motion for any given finger

Finger adduction:
Normal or good: little resistance
Fair: can adduct fingers toward middle finger but cannot hold against resistance
Poor: can adduct each finger tested through partial range of motion

Thumb abduction:
Normal to fair: completes range of motion with maximal to no resistance
Poor: completes partial range of motion
Trace: palpate belly of the abductor pollicis brevis in centre of the thenar eminence, medial to the opponens pollicis
None: no contractile activity |

Table 3.1 Cervical radiculopathy explorations (continued). Data from Giles [6] and Hislop & Montgomery [8].

Lumbar radiculopathy exploration

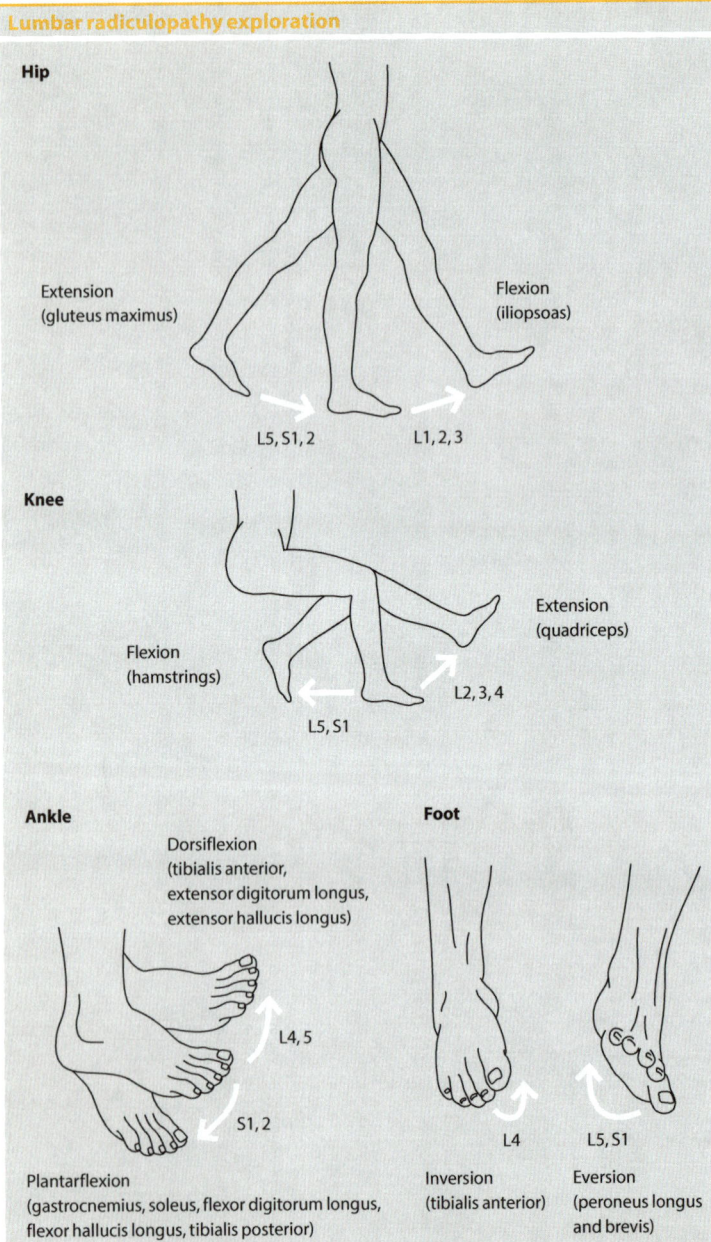

Figure 3.3 Lumbar radiculopathy exploration. Image adapted from Giles [7]. © 2009, Elsevier.

it up to the big toe. A positive Babinski sign consists of extension and separation of the toes, rather than flexion. Hyperreflexia (abnormally brisk reflexes), clonus, involuntary rhythmical muscle contractions and relaxations, are also abnormal responses to reflex testing.

Over recent years, several screening tools for distinguishing neuropathic from nociceptive pain have been validated (Table 3.3) [12]. Questionnaires (Neuropathic Pain Questionnaire) [13], ID PAIN [14] and PainDETECT [15], rely only on interview questions. The Leeds Assessment of Neuropathic Symptoms and Signs (LANSS) scale [16], Neuropathic Pain in 4 Questions (Douleur Neuropathique en 4 Questions; DN4) questionnaire [17] and the Standardized Evaluation of Pain (StEP) [18] use interview questions and physical tests (pinprick and tactile hypoaesthesia, pain to light touch) and achieve higher sensitivity and specificity than the screening tools that use only interview questions [12]. These tools can assist the practitioner to make a diagnosis of neuropathic pain.

How is sciatica classified?

Although the term 'sciatica' is simple and easy to use, it can be a confusing term [19]. For most researchers and clinicians, it refers to a radiculopathy involving one of the lower extremities, mostly related to disc herniation. As such, the term sciatica is too restrictive as nerve roots from L1 to L4 may also be involved in the same process. However, even more confusing is the fact that patients, and many clinicians alike, use sciatica to describe any pain arising from the lower back and radiating down to the leg [20].

Clinicians should conduct a focused history and physical examination to help place patients with low back pain (LBP) into one of three broad categories: nonspecific LBP, back pain potentially associated with spinal stenosis, or back pain potentially associated with another specific spinal cause [21]. Nonspecific lumbar pain (nonspecific mechanical LBP) is due to structural changes, postural or functional overload on the spinal column and its muscles or ligaments. It is diagnosed by excluding other processes. Pain worsens with movement or changes in position and does not radiate to the lower limbs; if it does, pain distribution is not radicular,

Lumbar radiculopathy explorations

Cervical nerve root	Pain	Motor weaknesses	Reflexes tested	Exam	Findings (response)
L4	Low back to hip to anterolateral thigh to medial leg	Extension of quadriceps	Quadriceps, tibialis anterior, extensor digitorum longus, extensor hallucis longus	Knee extension, ankle dorsiflexion, foot inversion	*Knee extension:* **Normal to fair:** completes available range of motion and holds end position with maximal to no resistance **Poor:** completes available range of motion **Trace:** contractile activity can be palpated in muscle through the tendon but no joint movement occurs **None:** no palpable contractile activity *Ankle dorsiflexion and foot inversion:* **Normal to fair:** completes range of motion with maximal to no resistance **Poor:** completes partial range of motion **Trace:** some muscle contractile activity but no joint movement **None:** no palpable contraction
L5	Hip to lateral thigh and leg to dorsum of foot and big toe	Dorsiflexion of great toe and foot	Gluteus maximus, hamstrings, tibialis anterior, extensor digitorum longus, extensor hallucis longus, peroneus longus and brevis	Hip extension, knee flexion, ankle dorsiflexion, foot eversion	*Hip extension:* **Normal to fair:** completes range of motion with maximal to no resistance **Poor:** completes range of extension motion in side–lying position **Trace:** palpable contraction of gluteus maximus or hamstrings but no visible joint movement **None:** no palpable contraction *Knee flexion:* **Normal to fair:** holds end range flexion position with maximal to no resistance **Poor:** completes available range of motion in side lying **Trace:** tendons become prominent, but no visible movement occurs **None:** no palpable contraction of the muscles and tendons do not stand out

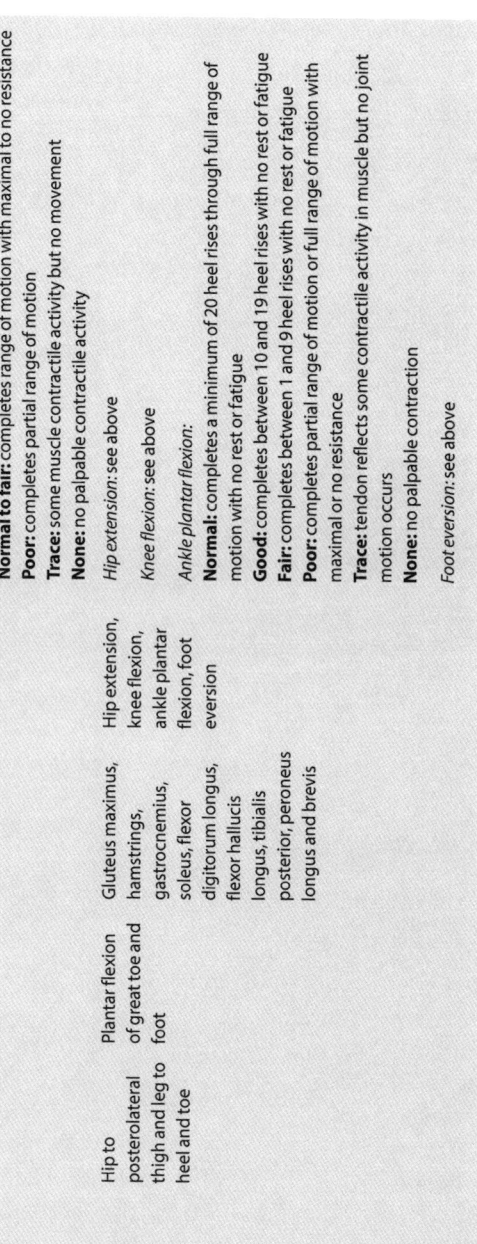

| S1 | Hip to posterolateral thigh and leg to heel and toe | Plantar flexion of great toe and foot | Gluteus maximus, hamstrings, gastrocnemius, soleus, flexor digitorum longus, flexor hallucis longus, tibialis posterior, peroneus longus and brevis | Hip extension, knee flexion, ankle plantar flexion, foot eversion | *Ankle dorsiflexion:* see above

Foot eversion:
Normal to fair: completes range of motion with maximal to no resistance
Poor: completes partial range of motion
Trace: some muscle contractile activity but no movement
None: no palpable contractile activity

Hip extension: see above

Knee flexion: see above

Ankle plantar flexion:
Normal: completes a minimum of 20 heel rises through full range of motion with no rest or fatigue
Good: completes between 10 and 19 heel rises with no rest or fatigue
Fair: completes between 1 and 9 heel rises with no rest or fatigue
Poor: completes partial range of motion or full range of motion with maximal or no resistance
Trace: tendon reflects some contractile activity in muscle but no joint motion occurs
None: no palpable contraction

Foot eversion: see above |

Table 3.2 Lumbar radiculopathy explorations. Data from Giles [6] and Hislop & Montgomery [8].

and therefore does not extend distally beyond the popliteal fossae. A recent work performed by Scholz and co-workers has demonstrated the importance of Lasègue's test in lumbar neuropathic pain [18].

Modern screening tools

Questionnaires	ID PAIN	NPQ	PainDETECT	LANSS	DN4	StEP
Symptoms reported						
Ongoing pain						−
Prickling, tingling, needles (any dysaesthesia)	+	+	+	+	+	+
Electric shocks or shooting	+	+	+	+	+	
Hot or burning	+	+	+	+	+	−
Numbness	+	+	+		+	
Pain evoked by light touching	+	+	+	+		
Painful cold or freezing pain		+			+	−
Pain evoked by mild pressure			+			
Pain evoked by heat or cold			+			
Pain evoked by changes in the weather		+				
Pain limited to joints	−					
Itching					+	
Temporal patterns or temporal summation						−
Radiation of pain						
Autonomic changes	+					
Physical examination						
Abnormal response to cold temperature (decrease or allodynia)						+
Hyperalgesia						+
Abnormal response to blunt pressure (decreased or evoked pain)						+
Decreased response to vibration						+
Brush allodynia				+	+	−
Raised soft touch threshold					+	−
Raised pinprick threshold				+	+	+
Straight leg raising test						+
Skin changes						−

Table 3.3 Modern screening tools. −, items that reduce the score. NPQ, Neuropathic Pain Questionnaire; LANSS, Leeds Assessment of Neuropathic Symptoms and Signs; DN4, Neuropathic Pain in 4 Questions (Douleur Neuropathique en 4 Questions); StEP, Standardized Evaluation of Pain. Data from Cruccu et al [12].

The characteristic clinical sign of spinal stenosis is pseudoclaudication, the neurogenic claudication of the lower limbs with bilateral (and often asymmetrical) pain symptoms, loss of sensitivity and/or weakness in the thighs and calves that is triggered by or worsens with walking and prolonged standing and improves upon decreasing lumbar lordosis (leaning forward, sitting or lying down). A differential diagnosis must be performed to exclude vascular claudication. For both neurogenic claudication and vascular claudication, the distance a patient can walk before symptoms appear is constant, but in the case of vascular claudication, pain does not improve with manoeuvres that decrease lumbar lordosis, and throbbing may be less intense or absent. Occasionally, in very advanced cases of spinal stenosis, the sacral roots are affected causing urinary and intestinal sphincter dysfunction and typical saddle anaesthesia (cauda equina syndrome). In these cases, rapid diagnosis and surgical treatment are essential in order to preserve sphincter function and prevent paraplegia. In most cases herniated discs are located below the emergence of the root at the intervertebral foramen, meaning that the root emerging from the foramen located immediately below the hernia is the most likely to be compressed. In other cases, however, the herniated disc enters the intervertebral foramen and compresses the root emerging at the same level. Therefore, a herniated disc may compress more than one nerve root. Final diagnosis is made based on clinical examination, combined potentially with additional tests. Medical imaging studies are indicated to exclude possible serious pathologies and to confirm the affected level in patients suffering lumbosacral radicular pain for longer than 3 months [22]. Given the considerable prevalence of herniated discs in asymptomatic patients, only results from imaging studies that fit the patient's clinical profile should be evaluated.

Examination begins as soon as the patient enters the room. The doctor will observe pain-free positions and walking habits (eg, limping, using a cane). The examination must check for any shoulder asymmetry, scoliosis, increase in lordosis, muscular atrophy and appearance of the skin (to rule out herpes zoster). The doctor should palpate the spinous apophyses, the paravertebral lumbar muscles, trochanters and sacroiliac joints and evaluate flexion, extension and lateral inclination movements.

Radicular pain radiates throughout the area innervated by the affected nerve root, which increases with movement, the Valsalva manoeuvre and stretching the nerve root in question. The most commonly used root stretch manoeuvres in use are as follows:

- Straight leg raising (SLR) test (Lasègue's sign): the clinician reproduces the radicular pain pattern by lifting the extended leg of a patient in a supine position. This test is useful in evaluating L5 and S1 radiculopathies. It has a sensitivity of 91% and a specificity of 26% [23].
- Bragard's sign: The clinician reproduces the radicular pain pattern by lifting the extended leg of a patient in supine position to just below the level for the SLR test while flexing the foot dorsally. Both the SLR and the Bragard tests are sensitive, but not very specific for radicular compression due to disc herniation.
- Crossed SLR test: when the clinician elevates the patient's extended, pain-free leg, it reproduces the radicular pain in the affected leg. This test for herniated disc-induced radiculopathy is very specific (88%), but less sensitive (29%) than the tests listed above [23].
- Reverse SLR: with the patient lying prone, the clinician extends the hip so that the leg is above table level with the knee flexed to reproduce radicular pain. This manoeuvre is useful for evaluating nerve roots L2, L3 and L4.

As mentioned earlier in this chapter, several screening tools for distinguishing neuropathic from nociceptive pain have been validated. PainDETECT was designed to detect neuropathic pain components in patients with LBP (reaches 80% sensitivity and specificity) [15]. The most recently developed screening tool to specifically evaluate patients with LBP is StEP (reaches 92% sensitivity and 97% specificity) [18].

What are the risk factors of low back pain chronicisation?

The clinical outlook for acute LBP is usually favourable; episodes tend to resolve in 2 weeks [24]. Nearly 90% of patients with acute LBP no longer require doctor's appointments within 3 months [25]. However, there are some risk factors or 'yellow flags' (see Table 2.3) that favour pain becoming chronic and producing long-term disability [26]. In recent conceptualisations of yellow flags, it has been suggested that their range of applicability should be confined primarily to psychological risk factors to differentiate them from other risk factors, such as social and environmental variables.

To systematically review the usefulness of individual risk factors or risk prediction instruments for identifying patients more likely to develop persistent disabling LBP, electronic searches of MEDLINE (1966–January 2010) and EMBASE (1974–February 2010) were performed, and the bibliographies of retrieved articles were reviewed to identify further articles. This review showed that the most helpful components for predicting persistent disabling LBP were maladaptive pain-coping behaviours, nonorganic signs, functional impairment, general health status and the presence of psychiatric comorbidities [27].

All guidelines mention psychosocial factors associated with poor prognosis with some describing them as 'yellow flags'. There is, however, considerable variation in the amount of details given about how to assess yellow flags or the optimal timing of the assessment. The Canadian and the New Zealand guidelines provide specific tools for identifying yellow flags and clear guidelines for what should be done once yellow flags are identified [28–30]. More recently, a randomised comparison of stratified primary care management for LBP (with or without radiculopathy) with current best practice has been reported [28]. This study demonstrated the benefits of targeted treatment that includes psychological therapy for patients at high risk of poor outcomes due to psychosocial issues. Patients were allocated into three risk groups, using the STarTBack screening tool [31,32]. In the intervention group, all medium-risk patients received standardised physiotherapy; in addition, high-risk patients received therapy to address physical symptoms and function, and psychosocial barriers to recovery. Patients in the control group received current best care. Compared with the control group, patients in the intervention group showed significant improvements in disability at 4 months and 12 months: benefits at 4 months were particularly marked in the high-risk patients.

How is radiated leg pain classified?

The most commonly affected intervertebral disc space is L4-L5, followed by L5-S1.

L1 radiculopathy

L1 radiculopathy is extremely rare. It leads to pain, paraesthesia and loss of sensitivity in the groin area and, on rare occasions, there may be a decrease in hip flexion strength. Deep tendon reflexes are normal. Differential diagnostic considerations include ilioinguinal and genitofemoral neuropathies. Physical examination may help distinguish between these conditions, but imaging of the lumbosacral spine or pelvis is often required [33].

L2 radiculopathy

Similar to L1 radiculopathy, L2 radiculopathy is also quite rare. It leads to pain, paraesthesia and loss of sensitivity in the anterolateral thigh with or without a decrease in hip flexion strength. Deep tendon reflexes are normal. Lateral femoral cutaneous neuropathy (meralgia paraesthetica) may mimic L2 radiculopathy; the presence of hip flexor weakness suggests radiculopathy rather than meralgia. Femoral neuropathy and upper lumbar plexopathy may present in a similar manner [33].

L3 radiculopathy

L3 radiculopathy is uncommon and leads to pain and paraesthesia in the inner thigh and knee. Examination shows weak hip flexion and adduction and weak knee extension (due to quadriceps and iliopsoas being affected) and decreased or absent patellar reflex. L3 radiculopathy may be confused with femoral neuropathy, obturator neuropathy, diabetic amyotrophy or upper lumbar plexopathy. Combined weakness of hip adduction and hip flexion differentiates L3 radiculopathy from femoral and obturator mononeuropathies [33].

L4 radiculopathy

L4 radiculopathy is common and leads to pain and paraesthesia in the inner thigh and sometimes the medial face of the leg. Weakening of the quadriceps (hip adduction and knee extension) and tibialis anterior muscles (foot dorsiflexion) may be observed. As with L3 radiculopathy, we may find decreased or absent patellar reflex. Lumbosacral plexopathy is the main differential diagnostic consideration; saphenous neuropathy is also a possibility in pure sensory syndromes [33].

L5 radiculopathy

L5 radiculopathy is very common and leads to pain in the buttock, posterolateral thigh, lateral face of the leg, lateral malleolus and, occasionally, the back of the foot. Paraesthesia in the lateral part of the leg and back of the foot may be observed. Examination shows weak dorsiflexion of the ankle (patients often present foot drop), foot inversion and eversion and extension of the big toe. In severe cases in which the gluteal muscles are affected, patients may experience weak leg abduction. We occasionally find hyperreflexia of the biceps femoris and posterior tibial reflex. Common peroneal neuropathy closely mimics and must be distinguished from L5 radiculopathy. Physical examination is helpful in localisation as weakness of foot eversion (mediated by the L5/peroneal-innervated peroneus muscles) in conjunction with inversion (mediated by the L5/tibial-innervated tibialis posterior) places the lesion proximal to the peroneal nerve. Lumbosacral plexopathy and sciatic neuropathy are important differential diagnostic considerations. The involvement of hip abductors (gluteus medius and minimus) indicates a lesion proximal to the sciatic nerve but does not differentiate L5 radiculopathy from lumbosacral plexopathy. Although there is no classic muscle stretch reflex true abnormality associated with L5 radiculopathy, an asymmetric internal hamstring reflex can support its presence [33].

S1 radiculopathy

S1 radiculopathy is the most common form of lumbar radiculopathy, it is associated with pain in the lower lumbar region, buttock, posterior thigh, calf and heel. Paraesthesia occurs along the back of the leg, lateral edge of the foot, heel, sole of the foot and, occasionally, the fourth and fifth toe. The most specific sign in an examination is weak plantar flexion due to weakness of the gastrocnemius or soleus muscle (patients experience difficulty walking on their toes). In addition, they present weak knee flexion and hip extension. Examination may also show a decreased or absent ankle-jerk reflex. Sciatic neuropathy and lower lumbosacral plexopathy may mimic S1 radiculopathy. Both of these conditions, however, also are expected to affect L5 innervated muscles [33].

References

1   Dionne CE, Dunn KM, Croft PR, et al. A consensus approach toward the standardization of back pain definitions for use in prevalence studies. *Spine*. 2008;33:95-103.

2   Merskey H, Bogduk N,eds. *Classification of Chronic Pain: Descriptions of Chronic Pain Syndromes and Definitions of Pain Terms*. Seattle, WA: IASP Press; 1994.

3   Misailidou V, Malliou P, Beneka A. Assessment of patients with neck pain: a review of definitions, selection criteria, and measurement tools. *J Chiro Med*. 2010;9:49-59.

4   Guzman J, Hurwitz EL, Carroll LJ, et al. A new conceptual model of neck pain. Linking onset, course, and care: the Bone and Joint Decade 2000-2010 Task Force on Neck Pain and its Associated Disorders. *Spine*. 2008;33:S14-S23.

5   Bogduk N, McGuirk B, eds. *Management of Acute and Chronic Neck Pain: An Evidence-Based Approach. Volume 13. Pain Research and Clinical Management*. 1st edn. Philadelphia, PA: Elsevier; 2006.

6   Giles LGF, ed. Cervical spine cases. In: *100 Challenging Spinal Pain Syndrome Cases*. Edinburgh, UK: Elsevier; 2009:219–223.

7   Giles LGF, ed. Lumbar spine cases. In: *100 Challenging Spinal Pain Syndrome Cases*. Edinburgh, UK: Elsevier; 2009:3-8.

8   Hislop HJ, Montgomery J. *Daniels and Worthingham's Muscle Testing: Techniques of Manual Examination*. 6th edn. Philadelphia, PA: W.B. Saunders Company; 1995.

9   Van Zundert J, Huntoon M, Patijn J, et al. Cervical radicular pain. *Pain Pract*. 2010;10:1-17.

10 Rubinstein SM, Pool JJ, van Tulder MW, Riphagen II, de Vet HC. A systematic review of the diagnostic accuracy of provocative tests of the neck for diagnosing cervical radiculopathy. *Eur Spine J*. 2007;16:307-319.

11 Chicuda H, Seichi A, Takesita K, et al. Correlation between pyramidal signs and the severity of cervical mielopathy. *Eur Spine J*. 2010;19:1684-1689.

12 Cruccu G, Truini A. Tools for assessing neuropathic pain. *PloS Med* 2009;6:1000045.

13 Leak AM, Cooper J, Dyer S, Williams KA, Turner-Stokes L, Frank AO. The Northwick Park Neck Pain Questionnaire devised to measure neck pain and disability. *Br J Rheumatol*. 1994;33:469-474.

14 Portenoy R. Development and testing of a neuropathic pain screening questionnaire: ID Pain. *Curr Med Res Opin*. 2006;22:1555-1565.

15 Freynhagen R, Baron R, Gockel U, Tölle TR. painDETECT: a new screening questionnaire to identify neuropathic components in patients with back pain. *Curr Med Res Opin*. 2006;22:1911-1920.

16 Bennett M. The LANSS Pain Scale: the Leeds Assessment of Neuropathic Symptoms and Signs. *Pain*. 2001;92:147-157.

17 Bouhassira D, Attal N, Alchaar H, et al. Comparison of pain syndromes associated with nervous or somatic lesions and development of a new neuropathic pain diagnostic questionnaire (DN4). *Pain*. 2005;114:29-36.

18 Scholz J, Mannion RJ, Hord DE, et al. A novel tool for the assessment of pain: validation in low back pain. *PLoS Med*. 2009;6:e1000047.

19 Fairbank JC. Sciatic: an archaic term. *Br Med J*. 2007;335:112.

20 Valat J-P, Genevay S, Marty M, et al. Sciatica. *Best Pract Res Clin Rheumatol*. 2010:24;241-252.

21 Chou R, Qaseem A, Snow V, et al. Diagnosis and treatment of low back pain: a joint clinical practice guideline from the American College of Physicians and the American Pain Society. *Ann Intern Med.* 2007;147:478-491.

22 Van Boxem K, Cheng J, Patijn J, et al. Lumbosacral radicular pain. *Pain Pract.* 2010;10:339-358.

23 Devillé WLJM, Windt DAWM, van der Dzaferagic A, et al. The test of Lasègue: systematic review of the accuracy in diagnosing herniated discs. *Spine.* 2000;25:1140-1147.

24 Pengel LHM, Herbert RD, Maher CG, Refshauge KM. Acute low back pain: a systematic review of its prognosis. *Br Med J.* 2003;327:323-325.

25 Croft PR, Macfarlane GJ, Papageorgiou AC, Thomas E, Silman AJ. Outcome of low back pain in general practice: a prospective study. *Br Med J.* 1998;316:1356-1359.

26 Guevara-López U, Covarrubias-Gómez A, Elías-Dob J, et al. Parámetros de prática para el manejo del dolor de espalda baja. *Cir Cir.* 2011;79:286-302.

27 Chou R, Shekelle P. Will this patient develop persistent disabling low back pain? *JAMA.* 2010;303:1295-1302.

28 Koes BW, van Tulder M, Lin CW, et al. An updated overview of clinical guidelines for the management of non-specific low back pain in primary care. *Eur Spine J.* 2010;19:2075-2094.

29 National Health Committee. New Zealand acute low back pain guide. Accident Rehabilitation & Compensation Insurance Corporation of New Zealand and the National Health Committee, Wellington, New Zealand; 2004.

30 Rossignol M, Arsenault B, Dionne C, et al. Clinic on Low-back pain in Interdisciplinary Practice (CLIP) guidelines. Available at: www.santpub-mtl.qc.ca/clip. Last accessed December 10, 2012.

31 Hill JC, Whitehurst DGT, Lewis M, et al. Comparison of stratified primary care management for low back pain with current best practice (STarTBack): a randomised controlled trial. *Lancet.* 2011;378:1560-1571.

32 Hill JC, Dunn KM, Lewis M, Mullis R, Main CJ, Foster NE, et al. A primary care back pain screening tool: identifying patient subgroups for initial treatment. *Arthritis Rheum.* 2008;59:632-641.

33 Tarulli AW, Raynor EM. Lumbosacral radiculopathy. *Neurol Clin.* 2007;25:387-405.

Development of this book was supported by funding from Pfizer

Chapter 4

How are the radiculopathies diagnosed?

Kees Vos

Clinical history to identify 'red flags' indicating possible serious spinal pathology

The first step in diagnosing sciatica and radicular pain is assessing the patient's clinical history, wherein the focus is on identifying so-called 'red flags', which may indicate an increased risk of serious pathology. A herniated disc is such a dominant reason for radiculopathic pain that all other possibly serious spinal pathologies should be ruled out [1].

It is important when taking a patient's history to obtain demographic information on the patient, for example age, sex, race and occupation, which can be useful to the physician in directing questioning. The physician needs to clarify if the reason for evaluation is primarily pain, numbness and tingling or weakness. The history of the present illness should include a thorough discussion of the pain and any previous similar symptoms. To quantify the pain, a numerical rating scale (0–10) or a visual analogue scale (0–100) can be used [2]. Specific information regarding the pain to be obtained while taking the patient's history includes:

- the intensity (ie, quality: sharp, dull or burning);
- location (back, buttock, hip, upper or lower leg or foot);
- onset (sudden or insidious) and factors associated with the onset (lifting, trauma, fall); and
- any remitting or exacerbating factors [3,4].

F. Laroche and S. Perrot (eds.), *Managing Sciatica and Radicular Pain in Primary Care Practice*, DOI: 10.1007/978-1-907673-56-6_4, © Springer Healthcare 2013

Other valuable information includes whether the symptoms are inter-mittent or constant, unilateral or bilateral, better or worse when in a particular position (sitting, standing, lying prone or lying supine) and, if worse, whether this is at a particular time of the day (issue of night pain) [5,6].

The mechanism of injury should be explored if the problem began suddenly. Knowing whether the injurious event involved flexion, exten-sion, lifting or twisting is valuable in gaining an understanding of the potential biomechanical issues involved. The onset of radicular pain often coincides with a movement involving flexion and rotation. When the cause of the injury is associated with trauma or work, details of the event are necessary [7]. Furthermore, information suggestive of a more severe neurological problem, such as progressive weakness, numbness and tingling or changes in bowel, bladder or sexual function, is essential. Noting any fevers or chills, night sweats and weight loss is particularly important in helping to rule out the potential of more severe pathology as the source of the symptoms and should expedite immediate further evaluation. Finally, information about previous evaluations, test results, medications and treatment interventions needs to be obtained [6]. Patients with herniated discs often have a long history of recurrent low back pain (LBP) prior to the onset of radicular symptoms [8].

Typically, the pain resulting from lumbosacral radiculopathy involves only one leg and radiation extends below the knee. The pain is localised in the dermatome of one of the lower back spinal nerve roots. Sometimes, the pain is located only in the lower leg and foot. The nature of the pain is sharp (stabbing, needling), can be clearly pointed out by the patient and often varies with the position of the body [9]. Reproduction of pain distally or pain that intensifies with coughing, sneezing or laughing, during a Valsalva manoeuvre or during any activity that increases intra-discal pressure, is suggestive of discogenic pain. A dermatomal distri-bution of pain, an increase in pain on coughing, sneezing or straining, paroxysmal pain and predominant leg pain are indicators of nerve root compression (Figure 4.1) [10].

Testing for lumbar nerve root compromise

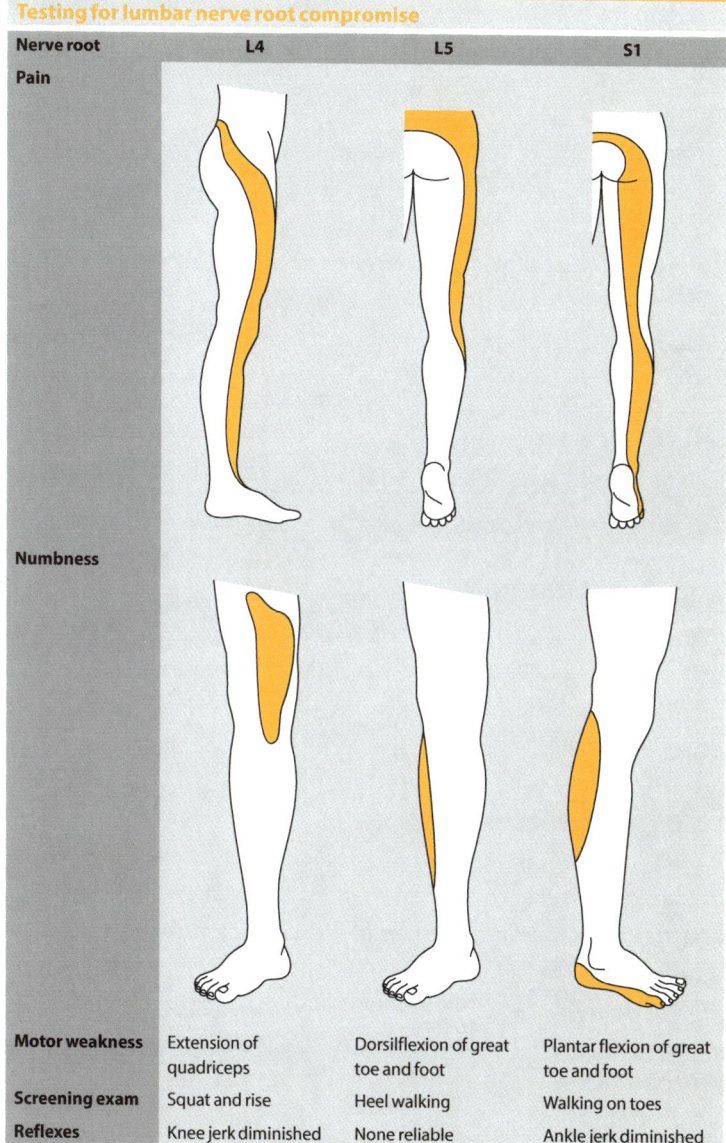

Nerve root	L4	L5	S1
Motor weakness	Extension of quadriceps	Dorsiflexion of great toe and foot	Plantar flexion of great toe and foot
Screening exam	Squat and rise	Heel walking	Walking on toes
Reflexes	Knee jerk diminished	None reliable	Ankle jerk diminished

Figure 4.1 Testing for lumbar nerve root compromise. Image adapted with permission from the Agency for Health Care Policy and Research [13].

The distinction between radicular and non-radicular ('referred' or 'somatic') pain is important. In practice this distinction is not always reliable. Features of non-radicular or referred pain are:

- more often in both legs;
- pain radiation not in accordance with the known dermatomes but diffusely spread over groins, hips, buttocks and posterior thigh;
- pain is not felt below knee level;
- the pain is of a dull nature and exact localisation of the pain is often difficult [11].

Pain in one leg is the dominating feature in lumbosacral radiculopathy. A typical history of sciatica has a fairly high sensitivity but uncertain specificity for herniated disc [10,12].

What is the duration of the pain?

The duration of the pain can be divided into an acute, sub-acute and chronic phase according to the International Association for the Study of Pain classification [14]. The acute phase lasts no longer than 3 weeks. The sub-acute phase is between 3 weeks and the start of the chronic phase at 3 months. Besides the 3 month period, there is another perhaps more appropriate definition of the chronic phase, namely 'pain without apparent biological value that has persisted beyond the normal tissue healing time' [15].

The primary care physician during history taking should be aware of the sometimes rare, serious causes of lumbosacral radicular pain. For example, think of such a rare cause in the case of atypical symptoms and signs that are not matching the usual pattern of radiculopathy. Alarm signals that may indicate a serious cause of LBP radiculopathy are shown in Table 4.1.

Assessment of pain severity using patient screening tools

In the assessment of pain and disability the use of disease-specific screening tools can be very helpful. The Roland Morris Disability Questionnaire (RMDQ) is an example of a commonly used tool [16,17]. Once radicular

Most common alarm signals in low back pain radiculopathy

- Patient is over 50 years of age when the complaint starts
- Ongoing pain independent of position or movement
- Increasing pain during the night
- Pain in both legs
- Extensive neurological deficits
- General feeling of weakness
- History of malignancy
- Unexplained weight loss

Table 4.1 Most common alarm signals in low back pain radiculopathy.

pain becomes chronic and the pain progressively changes towards a mixed pain of a dominant neuropathic nature, other screening tools are necessary. There are several symptom-based screening questionnaires developed for such a purpose. No single symptom is diagnostic of neuropathic pain, but combinations of certain symptoms, pain descriptors and findings from bedside test investigations increase the likelihood of a neuropathic pain condition [18].

Several verbal screening tools based on these signs and symptoms have been developed. They are simple and easy to use in clinical practice and may alert the physician to the need for careful examination in search of neuropathic pain, but they are no substitute for sound clinical judgement [19].

The full versions of the Leeds Assessment of Neuropathic Symptoms and Signs (LANSS) [20] and the Neuropathic Pain in 4 Questions (Douleur Neuropathique en 4 Questions; DN4) screening tools also include limited bedside sensory testing [21]. The painDETECT tool was originally developed to detect neuropathic disease components in patients with chronic LBP, but it is also useful for identifying other types of neuropathic pain [22].

Physical examination

A focused examination should at least include:

- the straight leg raising test (SLR); and
- neurologic examination that includes reflexes, muscle strength and the distribution of sensory symptoms.

Movement tests

The SLR is defined as the reproduction of the patient's sciatica between 30° and 70° of leg elevation [23]. The SLR test, which is also referred to as the Lasègue test, stresses the lower lumbar and upper sacral (L5 and S1) nerve roots [24]. During the SLR test, the patient is positioned in the supine position on the examination table. The physician then raises the leg to be tested by holding the heel with one hand and maintaining the ipsilateral knee in the fully extended position. The foot is then slowly raised from the table while maintaining the leg in a straight position until pain is elicited (Figure 4.2). The test can be further sensitised by adding neck flexion, internal rotation, adduction or dorsiflexion. When dorsiflexion is the sensitising manoeuvre, it is sometimes referred to as Bragard's sign.

Pain after 70° is more consistent with lumbar facet joint or sacroiliac pain. At 60° of elevation, a positive SLR has a high sensitivity for an L5-S1 radiculopathy. In a systematic review the pooled sensitivity was 0.91 (95% confidence interval [CI] 0.82–0.94), and pooled specificity was 0.26 (95% CI 0.16–0.38), with a positive predictive value of 81% [10,25]. The lower the angle, when the radicular pain is reproduced, the more specific the test [6].

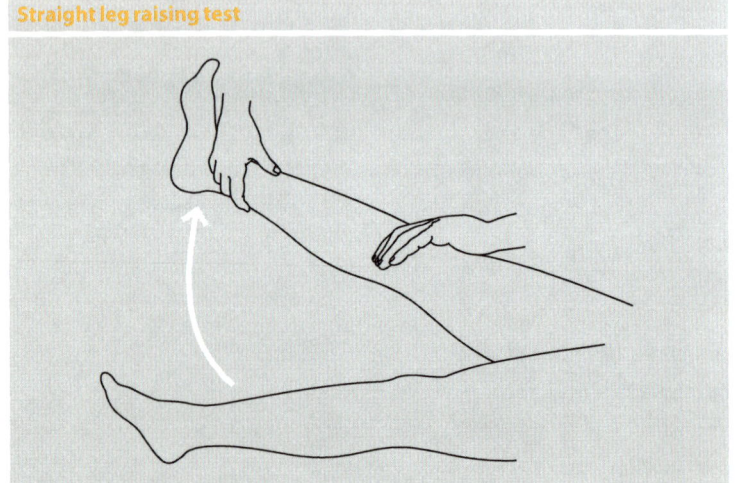

Straight leg raising test

Figure 4.2 Straight leg raising test. This test is also known as the Lasègue test.

The crossed SLR test (CSLR), which is also known as the well leg raise test, is performed by doing a SLR on the asymptomatic side. The CSLR test is positive if the patient has reproduction of his or her symptoms on the symptomatic side when the asymptomatic leg is raised. In the systematic review by Devillé et al, the CSLR was less sensitive 0.29 (95% CI 0.24–0.34), but more specific 0.88 (95% CI 0.86–0.90), with a positive predictive value of 98% [25]. A positive CSLR test often suggests a large herniation [26].

The femoral stress test, also known as the reversed Lasègue test (Figure 4.3), is performed with the patient prone and the anterior thigh fixed to the examination bed. Each knee is flexed in turn, stretching the femoral nerve roots in L2-L4. The test is positive if pain is felt in the anterior compartment of the thigh [1].

Sensory testing

As most disc herniations occur at L4-L5 or L5-S1, the cutaneous areas supplied by the respective nerves (L5 and S1) are the ones that most frequently demonstrate sensory changes. [27]. Although it can be helpful to evaluate light touch and temperature sensation, patients are best able to distinguish differences in sensation via pinprick testing or by means of

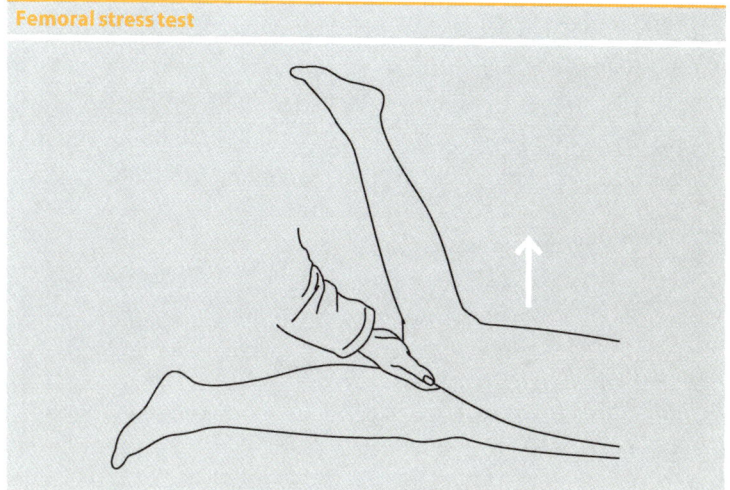

Femoral stress test

Figure 4.3 **Femoral stress test.** This test is also known as the reversed Lasègue test.

the von Frey hair test, or the vibration sense test using a 128-Hz tuning fork. By checking hyposensation in the medial (L4), dorsal (L5) and lateral or plantar (S1) aspects of the foot, the physician can screen for sensory changes in the nerve root distributions most likely to be affected.

Reflex testing

Because the S1 nerve is often affected due to the high incidence of L5-S1 disc herniations, a diminished Achilles reflex is one of the more common consequences of a radiculopathy observed during a clinical examination. Patellar (L3-L4), medial hamstring (L5) and Achilles (S1) reflexes should always be evaluated and compared to the contralateral side.

The medial hamstring reflex is elicited by tapping one of the medial hamstring tendons behind the knee, causing contraction of the tendon and flexion of the knee. The patient should be lying in the supine position with the knee and hip partially flexed and the leg supported by the examiner's hand.

Plantar stimulation (Babinski's test) and clonus testing are part of a comprehensive evaluation and, when positive, are indicators of upper motor neuron involvement [1].

Muscle testing

Muscle testing is most frequently graded according to the Oxford Scale, in which a grade of 0 is 'no movement' and a grade of 5 is 'normal' (Table 4.2) [28]. Muscle groups frequently evaluated include hip flexors (L2-L3), knee extensors (L3-L4), knee flexors (L5-S1), ankle dorsiflexors (L4-L5), plantarflexors (S1-S2) and the great toe extensor (L5). Subtle unilateral

The Oxford Scale for muscle testing	
Grade 0	No movement
Grade 1	Trace contraction without joint movement
Grade 2	Joint motion with gravity eliminated
Grade 3	Full range of motion against gravity alone
Grade 4	Complete movement of body part against gravity and some resistance
Grade 5	Normal

Table 4.2 The Oxford Scale for muscle testing. Data from Clarkson [28].

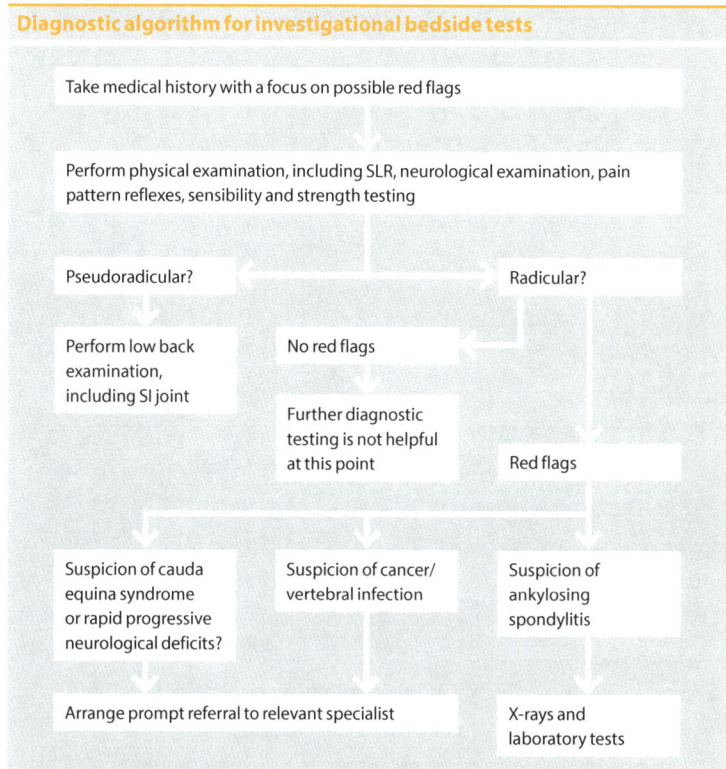

Figure 4.4 Diagnostic algorithm for investigational bedside tests. SI, Sacroiliac; SLR, straight leg raising test.

weakness in a myotome may lend support to the clinical diagnosis of radiculopathy. However, the Oxford Scale is not ideal for this purpose; since the examiner's arm strength is usually less than that of the patient's lower leg, the resistance test may miss subtle degrees of leg weakness.

Investigational bedside tests for diagnosis

The main component in the diagnosis of sciatica caused by disc herniation is the patient's history. The diagnostic value of reflex testing and sensory testing is limited due to poor reproducibility [12,29]. Few physical signs add useful additional information or result in the alteration of a diagnosis made on the basis of medical history [30,31] (Figure 4.4).

Summary of bedside testing
- Straight leg raise test, crossed straight leg raise test, femoral stress test.
- Reflex testing (patellar, achilles and Babinski's test).
- Sensory testing (light touch, temperature, pin prick, van Frey hair test, vibration sense test).
- Muscle testing (Oxford Scale).

What are the potential differential diagnoses?

In approximately 1% of patients with radiculopathy there are causes other than vertebral mechanical, for example, infection, tumour or fracture. The most important disorders to take into account when diagnosing radiculopathy are presented in Table 4.3. There are several causes of pseudoradicular pain such as peripheral neuropathy, myofascial syndromes, vascular diseases and osteoarthritis. Spondylarthropathies (eg, ankylosing spondylitis) should also be taken into consideration [32,33].

The most frequent finding in the cauda equina syndrome is urinary retention (90% sensitivity) [26]. In patients without urinary retention, the probability of the cauda equina syndrome is approximately 1 in 10,000 [23].

When diagnosing lumbar spinal stenosis, there is a tendency to focus on imaging studies, but there is a difference between the clinical and radiologic diagnosis of lumbar spinal stenosis. Therefore, clinical and radiologic findings should be considered together when diagnosing this condition [29].

In a large prospective study in a primary care setting, a history of cancer, unexplained weight loss, failure to improve after 1 month and age older than 50 years of age was each associated with a higher likelihood for cancer [34]. The probability of cancer in patients presenting with back pain increases from approximately 0.7% to 9% in patients with a history of cancer. In patients with any one of the other above three risk factors, the likelihood of cancer only increases slightly [34]. A review that assessed the accuracy of diagnosing LBP in nine studies concluded that the combination of history and erythrocyte sedimentation rate had a relatively high diagnostic accuracy in vertebral cancer [35].

Differential diagnostic considerations

Possible cause	Key features in patient history and physical examination
Cauda equina syndrome	Urinary retention
	Motor deficits at multiple levels
	Saddle anaesthesia
	Faecal incontinence
Ankylosing spondylitis (inflammatory back pain)	Morning stiffness more supple during the day
	Improvement with exercise
	Alternating buttock pain
	Awakening due to back pain during the second part of the night
	Younger age
Spinal stenosis	Radiating leg pain
	Older age
	Pseudoclaudication
Vertebral compression fracture	History of osteoporosis
	Use of corticosteroids
	Older age
Cancer	History of cancer with new onset of low back pain
	Unexplained weight loss
	Failure to improve after 1 month
	Age over 50 years
Severe/progressive neurologic deficits	Progressive motor weakness

Table 4.3 Differential diagnostic considerations. Data from Chou et al [23].

A study in the US on the diagnosis and treatment of LBP in primary care found that 4% of patients had a compression fracture, 3% spondylolisthesis, 0.7% had a tumour or metastasis, 0.3% ankylosing spondylitis and 0.01% an infection [36].

When should imaging be used?

Plain radiographs are generally used as a starting point for imaging evaluation. In general, the course of acute lumbosacral radicular pain is favourable and plain radiographs are therefore not necessary during the first 4 to 6 weeks following initial assessment [23,31,37,38]. The correlation between symptoms and X-ray findings is poor, and so the chance of finding serious disease that is not suspected clinically is extremely low.

Despite this, referring for X-rays in order to gain reassurance is common-place in primary care. Such reassurance may be misplaced, as lumbar spine radiography is relatively insensitive to important diagnoses such as malignancy or infection at an early stage, which would be detected by other imaging techniques such as magnetic resonance imaging (MRI) [39]. Additionally, radiography of the lumbar spine in primary care patients with LBP of at least 6 weeks' duration is not associated with improved patient functioning, severity of pain or overall health status, but is associated with an increase in doctor workload [40] and overall healthcare costs. Most patients with LBP need an explanation of the causes and treatments rather than roentgenograms [41].

MRI is generally considered the optimal modality for spinal imaging, especially when disc or radicular pathology is suspected [23,42]; however, computed tomography (CT) can also be useful [42]. The imaging algorithm choice for an imaging study may be determined by what is available to the clinician and patient contraindications for an MRI study. The availability of CT scans and MRI's differs between countries and even within countries.

For various reasons, CT or CT myelography have been relegated to a secondary role in the imaging evaluation of the spine. CT scanning is inferior to MRI in showing a discus herniation, CT myelographic studies are more complex and bear a higher risk of allergic complications, intramedullar infection and spinal fluid leakage. Furthermore, CT scans involve significantly higher radiation exposure than X-rays or MRI scans, which may impact on the patient's long-term health.

Although early use of imaging, whether by MRI, CT or X-ray, is associated with greater early pain reduction it does not affect overall treatment outcome and so may not justify the additional costs involved [43,44].

However, diagnostic imaging should be performed at short notice when there are severe and progressive neurological deficits or if the medical history uncovers any 'red flags' such as fevers, unexplained weight loss, night pain or bladder changes, which suggest the potential for more severe, underlying pathology. MRI should also be considered when a diagnosis of spinal malignancy, infection, fracture, cauda equina syndrome or ankylosing spondylitis or other inflammatory disorders is suspected.

A large protruding hernia on L4-L5 as seen on magnetic resonance image

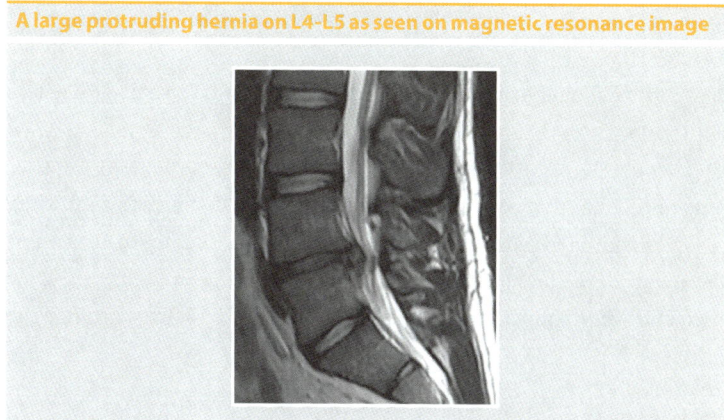

Figure 4.5 A large protruding hernia on L4-L5 as seen on magnetic resonance image.

MRI is also the most appropriate next step when the course of the suspected herniated disc is unfavourable and surgery becomes a possibility. Bear in mind that disc herniation is highly prevalent (20–36%) in people without symptoms and who do not have sciatica [31,45]. Therefore in the clinical judgment of MRI results it is important to be aware that there is a high proportion of asymptomatic discus protrusions (Figure 4.5). Sensitivity and specificity values of MRI in the diagnosis of disc herniation range from 71–100% and 50–86%, respectively [30]. If there is no favourable outcome for the patient after 6–8 weeks, then specialist referral is indicated.

Electrodiagnostic testing

Electrodiagnostic evaluation is not required in every patient with a suspected radiculopathy. When the results of the imaging study do not match the clinical findings, electromyography (EMG) can be valuable in assessing for radiculopathy and to differentiate from other neuropathies, especially polyneuropathy [6]. Electrodiagnostic testing may be used to assist in surgical decision making, especially by identifying the anatomic level of nerve injury when multiple levels are involved and when motor deficiency is observed.

Patient referrals – who should be referred and when?

The patient should be referred to a neurologist, pain specialist or, where appropriate, to a rheumatologist, for further diagnostic assessment when their general practitioner suspects a serious or rare cause of sciatica. Urgent referral to a neurosurgeon for decompression is indicated when a cauda equina syndrome is suspected. Referral to a neurosurgeon or neurologist is also indicated for assessment in the case of uncontrollable pain and when there is insufficient improvement 6 to 8 weeks after the initial visit [1,23,35,37].

References

1   Mens JMA, Chavannes AW, Koes BW, et al. NHG-Standaard lumbosacraal radiculair syndroom [NHG Guideline on lumbosacral radicular syndrome]. *Huisarts Wetenschap*. 2005;48:171-178.

2   Maughan EF, Lewis JS. Outcome measures in chronic low back pain. *Eur Spine J*. 2010;19:1484-1494.

3   Sriwatanakul K, Kelvie W, Lasagna L, et al. Studies with different types of visual analog scales for measurement of pain. *Clin Pharmacol Ther*. 1983;34:234-239.

4   von Korff M, Jensen MP, Karoly P. Assessing global pain severity by self-report in clinical and health services research. *Spine*. 2000;25:3140-3151.

5   Andersson GB. Diagnostic considerations in patients with back pain. *Phys Med Rehab Clin N Am*. 1998;9:309-322.

6   Smeal WL, Tyburski M, Alleva J. Discogenic/radicular pain. *Dis Mon*. 2004;50:636-669.

7   Miranda H, Viikari-Juntura E, Martikainen R, et al. Individual factors, occupational loading, and physical exercise as predictors of sciatic pain. *Spine*. 2002;27:1102-1109.

8   Deyo RA, Loeser JD, Bigos SJ. Herniated lumbar intervertebral disk. *Ann Intern Med*. 1990;15:598-603.

9   Picavet HS, Schouten JS. Physical load in daily life and low back problems in the general population: the MORGEN study. *Prev Med*. 2000;31:506-512.

10   Vroomen PC, de Krom MC, Knottnerus JA. Diagnostic value of history and physical examination in patients suspected of sciatica due to disc herniation: a systematic review. *J Neurol*. 1999;246:899-906.

11   Waddell G. *The Back Pain Revolution*. Edinburgh, UK: Churchill Livingstone; 1999.

12   van den Hoogen HM, Koes BW, van Eijk JT, Bouter LM. On the accuracy of history, physical examination, and erythrocyte sedimentation rate in diagnosing low back pain in general practice. A criteria-based review of the literature. *Spine*. 1995;20:318-327.

13   Agency for Health Care Policy and Research. Quick Reference Guide Number 14: Acute low back problems in adults: assessment and treatment. Available at: www.ncbi.nlm.nih.gov/books/NBK52134/. Accessed August 23, 2012.

14   Merskey H, Bogduk N. *Classification of Chronic Pain*. 2nd edn. Seattle, WA: IASP Press; 1994.

15   Harstall C, Ospina M. How prevalent is chronic pain? *IASP Pain: Clinical Updates* 2003;11:1-4.

16   Ostelo RWJG, de Vet HCW, Knol DL, van den Brandt PA. 24-item Roland Morris Disability Questionnaire was preferred out of six functional status questionnaires for post-lumbar disc surgery. *J Clin Epidemiol*. 2004;57:268-276.

17   Beurskens AJ, de Vet HC, Koke AJ. Responsiveness of functional status in low back pain: a comparison of different instruments. *Pain*. 1996;65:71-76.

18 Cruccu G, Anand P, Attal N, et al. EFNS guidelines on neuropathic pain assessment. *Eur J Neur* 2004;11: 13-62.

19 Haanpää, ML, Backonja MM, Bennet MI, et al. Assessment of neuropathic pain in primary care. *Am J Medicine* 2009;122:S13–S21.

20 Bennett M. The LANSS Pain Scale: the Leeds assessment of neuropathic symptoms and signs. *Pain.* 2001;92:147-157.

21 Bouhassira D, Attal N, Alchaar H, et al. Comparison of pain syndromes associated with nervous or somatic lesions and development of a new neuropathic pain diagnostic questionnaire (DN4). *Pain.* 2005;114:29-36.

22 Freynhagen R, Baron R, Gockel U, Tölle TR. painDETECT: a new screening questionnaire to identify neuropathic components in patients with back pain. *Curr Med Res Opin.* 2006;22:1911-1920.

23 Chou R, Qaseem A, Snow V, et al. Diagnosis and treatment of low back pain: a joint clinical practice guideline from the American College of Physicians and the American Pain Society. *Ann Intern Med.* 2007;147:478-491.

24 Lauder TD. Physical examination signs, clinical symptoms, and their relationship to electrodiagnostic findings and the presence of radiculopathy. *Phys Med Rehab Clin N Am.* 2002;13:451-467.

25 Devillé WL, van der Windt DA, Dzaferagić A, Bezemer PD, Bouter LM. The test of Lasègue: systematic review of the accuracy in diagnosing herniated discs. *Spine.* 2000;25:1140-1147.

26 Saal JA. Natural history and nonoperative treatment of lumbar disc herniation. *Spine.* 1996;21:2S-9S.

27 Kortelainen P, Puranen J, Koivisto E, Lähde S. Symptoms and signs of sciatica and their relation to the localization of the lumbar disc herniation. *Spine.* 1985;10:88-92.

28 Clarkson HM. *Musculoskeletal Assessment: Joint Range of Motion and Manual Muscle Strength.* Philadelphia: Lippincott Williams & Wilkins; 2000.

29 de Graaf I, Prak A, Bierma-Zeinstra S, Thomas S, Peul W, Koes B. Diagnosis of lumbar spinal stenosis: a systematic review of the accuracy of diagnostic tests. *Spine.* 2006;31:1168-1176.

30 Vroomen PC, de Krom MC, Knottnerus JA. Consistency of history taking and physical examination in patients with suspected lumbar nerve root involvement. *Spine.* 2000;25:91-96.

31 Valat JP, Genevay S, Marty M, Rozenberg S, Koes B. Sciatica. *Best Pract Res Clin Rheumatol.* 2010;24:241-252.

32 Rudwaleit M, Metter A, Listing J, Sieper J, Braun J. Inflammatory back pain in ankylosing spondylitis: a reassessment of the clinical history for application as classification and diagnostic criteria. *Arthritis Rheum.* 2006;54:569-578.

33 Mansour M, Cheema GS, Naguwa SM, et al. Ankylosing spondylitis: a contemporary perspective on diagnosis and treatment. *Semin Arthritis Rheum.* 2007;36:210-223.

34 Deyo RA, Diehl AK. Cancer as a cause of back pain: frequency, clinical presentation, and diagnostic strategies. *J Gen Intern Med.* 1988;3:230-238.

35 van Tulder M, Becker A, Bekkering T, et al. European guidelines for the management of acute non-specific low back pain in primary care. *Eur Spine J.* 2006;15:S169-S191.

36 Koes BW, van Tulder MW, Thomas S. Diagnosis and treatment of low back pain. *BMJ.* 2006;17:1430-1434.

37 NICE Clinical Guideline 88. Low back pain: early management of persistent non-specific low back pain. 2009. Available at http://publications.nice.org.uk/low-back-pain-cg88. Accessed August 23, 2012.

38 Hagen KB, Hilde G, Jamtvedt G, Winnem MF. The Cochrane review of bed rest for acute low back pain and sciatica. *Spine.* 2000;25:2932-2939.

39 Kendrick D, Fielding K, Bentley E, Miller P, Kerslake R, Pringle M. The role of radiography in primary care patients with low back pain of at least 6 weeks duration: a randomised (unblinded) controlled trial. *Health Technol Assess.* 2001;5:1-69.

40 Kendrick D, Fielding K, Bentley E, Kerslake R, Miller P, Pringle M. Radiography of the lumbar spine in primary care patients with low back pain: randomised controlled trial. *BMJ.* 2001;322:400-405.

41 Deyo RA, Diehl AK, Rosenthal M. Reducing roentgenography use. Can patient expectations be altered? *Arch Intern Med*. 1987;147:141-145.

42 Jarvik JG. Imaging of adults with low back pain in the primary care setting. *Neuroimaging Clin N Am*. 2003;13:293-305.

43 Gilbert FJ, Grant AM, Gillan MG, et al. Scottish Back Trial Group. low back pain: influence of early MR imaging or CT on treatment and outcome--multicenter randomized trial. *Radiology*. 2004;231:343-351.

44 Jarvik JG, Hollingworth W, Martin B, et al. Rapid magnetic resonance imaging vs radiographs for patients with low back pain: a randomized controlled trial. *JAMA*. 2003;289:2810-2818.

45 Buirski G, Silberstein M. The symptomatic lumbar disc in patients with low-back pain. Magnetic resonance imaging appearances in both a symptomatic and control population. *Spine*. 1993;18:1808-1811.

Development of this book was supported by funding from Pfizer

Chapter 5

What guidelines are available for sciatica and radicular pain?

Paolo Marchettini

Guidelines for the management of low back pain (LBP) and lumbar or cervical radiculopathy resulting from sciatica and other radicular pain syndromes have been published by a number of organisations, including:

- the European Commission Research Directorate General [1,2] from the COST B13 Working Group;
- the UK Royal College of General Practitioners (RCGP) [3] and the National Institute for Health and Clinical Excellence (NICE) [4];
- the Dutch College of General Practice [5];
- the American College of Physicians and the American Pain Society (ACP/APS) [6–8]; and
- the North American Spine Society (NASS) [9].

Most of the sciatica and LBP guidelines are aimed at primary care physicians, reflecting the fact that most patients with sciatica are treated in the primary care setting [10,11]. However, in many cases these guidelines relate to the management of nonspecific back pain, rather than sciatica due to radiculopathy. Indeed, the treatment guidelines published by the European Commission Research Directorate General [1,2] and NICE [4] specifically exclude pain of radicular origin.

A further limitation to all the guidelines is their failure to mention that several non-opioid agents (pregabalin, gabapentin and capsaicin) are now approved specifically for the treatment of neuropathic pain.

F. Laroche and S. Perrot (eds.), *Managing Sciatica and Radicular Pain in Primary Care Practice*, DOI: 10.1007/978-1-907673-56-6_5, © Springer Healthcare 2013

These agents may have a useful place in the management of patients for whom non-steroidal anti-inflammatory drugs (NSAIDs) are insufficient, before opioid therapy is considered.

Dutch College of General Practice guidelines

The guidelines of the Dutch College of General Practice are among the few guidelines that specifically address the management of sciatica resulting from radiculopathy, rather than nonspecific LBP [5,11]. The principal recommendations of these guidelines are shown in Table 5.1 [5,11]. They emphasise that the diagnosis of sciatica is based on the medical history and physical examination, after excluding specific 'red flag' signs or symptoms (see Chapter 4); imaging procedures such as magnetic resonance imaging (MRI) or computed tomography (CT) are not indicated. However, relevant red flags such as urinary disturbances (indicating cauda equina involvement), fever and increased erythrocyte sedimentation rate (indicating infection) and worsening of pain while lying in bed (indicating metastasis) are not included. The Dutch guidelines focus on the lower lumbar and the cervical roots, and the Wassermann manoeuvre for the diagnosis of L3-L4 radiculopathy is not mentioned. Initial management is conservative and includes patient education, encouragement of physical activity and appropriate analgesia. Patients whose symptoms do not improve after 6 to 8 weeks of conservative management should be referred to an appropriate consultant, such as a rheumatologist or neurologist.

UK Royal College of General Practitioners guidelines

The UK RCGP guidelines [3] relate to the management of acute LBP and they recommend diagnostic triage to distinguish between:

- simple backache (nonspecific LBP);
- nerve root pain; and
- possible serious spinal pathology.

Treatment recommendations focus primarily on simple backache and, as in the Dutch guidelines, the emphasis is on conservative management. Paracetamol is recommended as first-line drug therapy, with NSAIDs being substituted in patients for whom paracetamol does not provide adequate pain relief; however, the guidelines note that NSAIDs are less effective in patients with nerve root pain than in those with simple backache [3]. A short course (<1 week) of muscle relaxants such as diazepam can be

Recommendations of the Dutch College of General Practice guidelines for the diagnosis and treatment of sciatica

Diagnosis

Exclude 'red flag' conditions such as malignancy, osteoporotic fractures, radiculitis and cauda equina syndrome.

Take a history to determine:
- the localisation and severity of the pain;
- loss of strength;
- sensory disorders;
- duration;
- course;
- influence of coughing, rest or movement; and
- consequences for daily activities.

Perform a physical examination, including neurological testing, eg a straight leg raising test (Lasègues sign).

Carry out the following tests in patients with a dermatomal pattern, positive Lasègue's sign, loss of strength or sensory disorders:
- Achilles or knee tendon reflexes;
- sensitivity of lateral and medial sides of feet and toes;
- strength of big toe during extension;
- walking on toes and heel (left-right differences); and
- crossed Lasègue's sign.

Imaging or laboratory diagnostic tests are only indicated in red flag conditions and are not useful in cases of suspected disc herniation.

Treatment

Explain the cause of the symptoms and reassure the patient that symptoms usually diminish over time without specific treatment.

Advise the patient to stay active and continue their daily activities: a few hours of bed rest may relieve symptoms, but does not result in faster recovery.

If necessary, prescribe analgesia according to a four-step schedule:
- paracetamol;
- nonsteroidal anti-inflammatory drugs (NSAIDs);
- tramadol, paracetamol or NSAID in combination with codeine; and
- morphine.

Refer to a neurosurgeon immediately in cases of cauda equina syndrome or acute severe paresis or progressive paresis (within a few days).

Refer to a neurologist, rheumatologist or orthopaedic surgeon for consideration of surgery in cases of intractable radicular pain (not responsive to morphine), or if pain does not diminish after 6–8 weeks of conservative management.

Table 5.1 Recommendations of the Dutch College of General Practice guidelines for the diagnosis and treatment of sciatica. Data from Mens et al [5] and Koes et al [10].

considered if neither paracetamol nor NSAIDs provide sufficient pain relief. Narcotics such as morphine or pethidine should be avoided as much as possible and their use limited to a maximum of 2 weeks.

American College of Physicians and the American Pain Society guidelines

The ACP and APS have published joint guidelines for the diagnosis and treatment of LBP, including pain due to radiculopathy [6]. These guidelines were derived from systematic reviews of the evidence for the benefits and risks of pharmacological [7] and nonpharmacological [8] therapies in patients with acute or chronic LBP (cLBP). They make seven recommendations (Table 5.2), most of which are considered to be strong recommendations based on moderate-quality evidence (a strong recommendation indicates that the benefits of a particular indication clearly outweigh the risks [6]).

These guidelines emphasise that a focused history and physical examination should be performed in all patients with LBP, in order to distinguish between:

- back pain potentially associated with radiculopathy or spinal stenosis;
- back pain potentially associated with other specific spinal causes; or
- nonspecific LBP.

In common with the Dutch guidelines, the ACP/APS guidelines emphasise that patients with persistent LBP and suspected radiculopathy should not routinely undergo imaging because there is no evidence that routine imaging improves treatment outcomes [6,12]. However, imaging (preferably by MRI) should be performed in patients with persistent pain in whom surgery or epidural steroid injections are being considered.

As in the Dutch guidelines, the ACP/APS guidelines recommend conservative management, aimed at promoting continued activity and self-care. Appropriate analgesia can be used, depending on the relative benefits and risks in each individual patient; paracetamol (acetaminophen) and NSAIDs are recommended as first-line treatment. The ACP/ASP guidelines differ from the Dutch guidelines in that nonpharmacological therapies, such as spinal manipulation for acute LBP, or exercise therapy, acupuncture or massage therapy for chronic or subacute LBP, are recom-

Recommendations from the American College of Physicians and the American Pain Society guidelines for the diagnosis and treatment of low back pain

Diagnosis

A focused history should be obtained, and a physical examination performed, to categorise the cause of LBP:

- nonspecific LBP;
- back pain potentially associated with radiculopathy or spinal stenosis; or
- back pain potentially associated with another specific spinal cause.

The history should include an assessment of psychosocial risk factors, which are predictive of the risk of chronic disabling back pain.

Imaging or other diagnostic tests should not be performed routinely in patients with nonspecific LBP.

Diagnostic imaging and testing should be performed in patients with LBP when severe or progressive neurologic deficits are present, or when serious underlying conditions are suspected on the basis of the history and physical examination. Patients with persistent LBP and signs or symptoms of radiculopathy or spinal stenosis should undergo imaging (preferably with MRI) only if they are potential candidates for surgery or epidural steroid injection.

Treatment

Patients should be provided with evidence-based information on LBP with regard to their expected course, advised to remain active and provided with information about effective self-care options.

For patients with LBP, medications proven to be beneficial should be used in conjunction with back care information and self-care; the severity of baseline pain and functional deficits, the potential benefits, risks, relative lack of long-term efficacy and safety data should be considered before initiating therapy. First-line medication should consist of paracetamol or NSAIDs in most cases.

For patients who do not improve with conservative management, the addition of nonpharmacological therapies with proven benefits should be considered*:

- For acute LBP, spinal manipulation can be considered.
- For chronic or subacute LBP, options include intensive interdisciplinary rehabilitation, exercise therapy, acupuncture, massage therapy, spinal manipulation, yoga, cognitive-behavioural therapy or progressive relaxation.

Table 5.2 Recommendations from the American College of Physicians and the American Pain Society guidelines for the diagnosis and treatment of low back pain. *This is considered a weak recommendation, indicating that the benefits of these interventions have not been clearly shown to outweigh the benefits. LBP, low back pain. Data from Mens et al [5].

mended in patients who do not benefit from initial conservative therapy. However, this is considered a weak recommendation, based on moderate-quality evidence, which indicates that the benefits of these therapies have not been clearly shown to outweigh the risks [6].

The ACP/APS guidelines include algorithms for the diagnosis (Figure 5.1) and subsequent management (Figure 5.2) of LBP [6].

American College of Physicians and the American Pain Society guidelines on the diagnosis of low back pain

Adults with LBP

Perform a focused history and physical examination, evaluating:
- Duration of symptoms
- Risk factors for potentially serious conditions
- Symptoms suggesting radiculopathy or spinal stenosis
- Presence and severity of neurologic deficits
- Psychosocial risk factors

(Recommendation 1)

Are any potentially serious conditions strongly suspected? (see Diagnostic work-up) (Recommendation 2)

Yes

No

Perform diagnostic studies to identify cause (see Diagnostic work-up) (Recommendation 2)

No

Specific causes identified?

Yes

Back pain is mild with no substantial functional impairment?

Yes

Advise about self-care

Review indications for reassessment

(Recommendation 5)

No

Advise about self-care (Recommendation 5)

Discuss noninvasive treatment options:
- Pharmacologic (Recommendation 6)
- Nonpharmacologic (Recommendation 7)

Treat specific cause as indicated, consider consultation

Arrive at a shared decision regarding therapy trial. Educate patient

Patient accepts risks and benefit of therapy?

Yes

Specific causes identified?

Yes

No

No

Continue self-care
Reassess in 1 month

Go to Figure 5.2, 'LBP not on therapy'

Go to Figure 5.2, 'LBP on therapy'

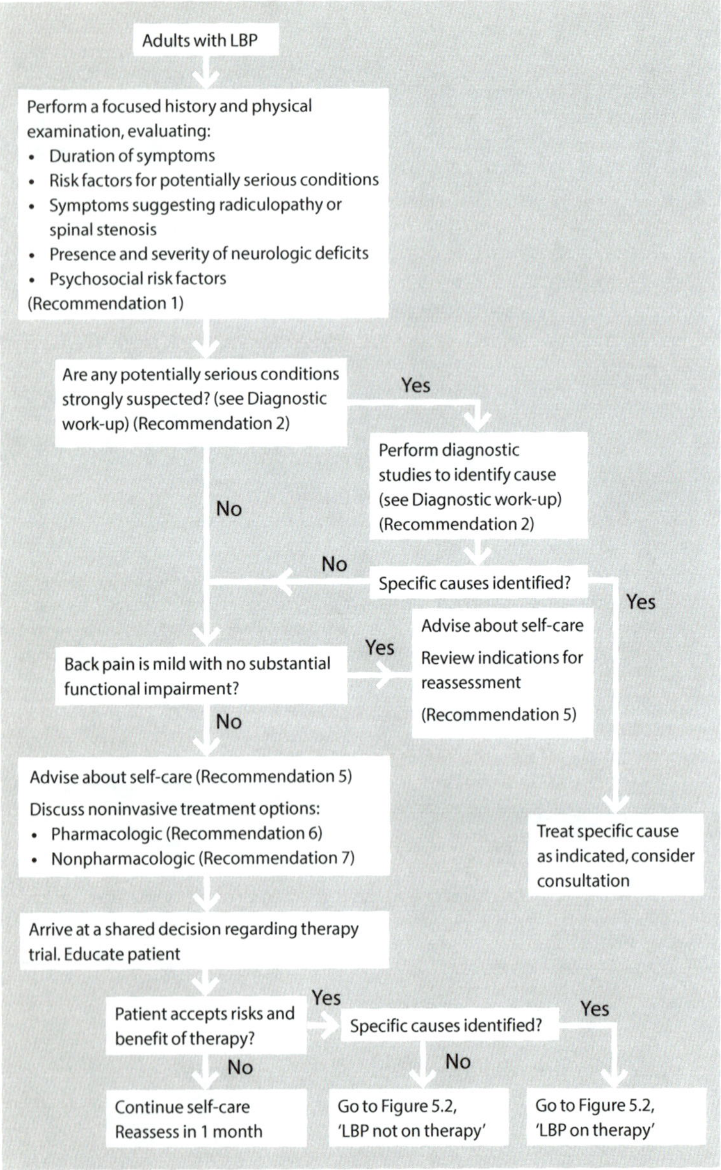

Figure 5.1 American College of Physicians and the American Pain Society guidelines on the diagnosis of low back pain (continues opposite).

American College of Physicians and the American Pain Society guidelines on the diagnosis of low back pain (continued)

Diagnostic work-up

Possible cause	Key features on history or physical examination	Imaging*	Additional studies*
Cancer	History of cancer with new onset of LBP	MRI	ESR
	Unexplained weight loss Failure to improve after 1 month Age >50 years	Lumbosacral plain radiography	
	Multiple risk factors present	Plain radiography or MRI	
Vertebral infection	Fever Intravenous drug use Recent infection	MRI	ESR and/or CRP
Cauda equina syndrome	Urinary retention Motor deficits at multiple levels Faecal incontinence Saddle anaesthesia	MRI	None
Vertebral compression fracture	History of osteoporosis Use of corticosteroids Older age	Lumbosacral plain radiography	None
Ankylosing spondylitis	Morning stiffness Improvement with exercise Alternating buttock pain Awakening due to back pain during the second part of the night Younger age	Anterior-posterior pelvis plain radiography	ESR and/or CRP, HLA-827
Severe/progressive neurologic deficits	Progressive motor weakness	MRI	Consider EMG/NCV
Herniated disc (Recommendation 4)	Back pain with leg pain in an L4, L5 or S1 nerve root distribution Positive SLR test or crossed SLR test	None	None
	Symptoms present >1 month	MRI	Consider EMG/NCV
Spinal stenosis (Recommendation 4)	Radiating leg pain Older age (Pseudoclaudication a week predictor)	None	None
	Symptoms present >1 month	MRI	Consider EMG/NCV

*Level of evidence for diagnostic evaluation is variable

Figure 5.1 American College of Physicians and the American Pain Society guidelines on the diagnosis of low back pain (continued). This algorithm must not be used for back pain associated with major trauma, nonspinal back pain or back pain due to systemic illness. CRP, C-reactive protein; EMG, electromyography; ESR, erythrocyte sedimentation rate; LBP, low back pain; MRI, magnetic resonance imaging; NCV, nerve conduction velocity; SLR, straight leg raising. Data from Chou et al [6].

American College of Physicians and the American Pain Society guidelines on the diagnosis of low back pain

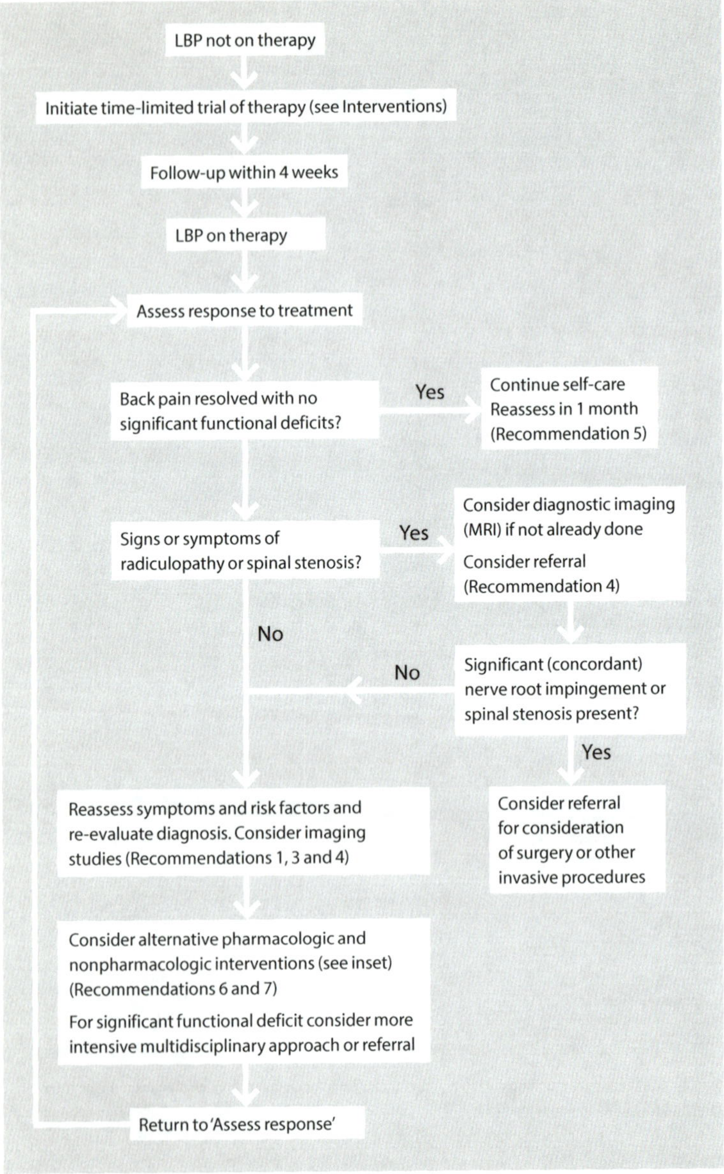

Figure 5.2 American College of Physicians and the American Pain Society guidelines on the diagnosis of low back pain (continues opposite).

American College of Physicians and the American Pain Society guidelines on the diagnosis of low back pain (continued)

Interventions (Recommendations 5, 6 and 7)

		Type of LBP and duration	
		Acute <4 weeks	Subacute or chronic >4 weeks
Self-care	Advice to remain active	✓	✓
	Books, handout	✓	✓
	Application of superficial heat	✓	
Pharmacologic therapy	Acetaminophen	✓	✓
	NSAIDs	✓	✓
	Skeletal muscle relaxants	✓	
	Antidepressants (TCA)		✓
	Benzodiazepines	✓	✓
	Tramadol, opioids	✓	✓
Nonpharmacologic therapy	Spinal manipulation	✓	✓
	Exercise therapy		✓
	Massage		✓
	Acupuncture		✓
	Yoga		✓
	Cognitive-behavioural therapy		✓
	Progressive relaxation		✓
	Intensive interdisciplinary rehabilitation		✓

*Interventions supported by grade B evidence (at least fair-quality evidence of moderate benefit, or small benefit but no significant harms, costs or burdens). No intervention was supported by grade A evidence (good-quality evidence of substantial benefit).

Figure 5.2 American College of Physicians and the American Pain Society guidelines on the diagnosis of low back pain (continued). This algorithm must not be used for back pain associated with major trauma, nonspinal back pain or back pain due to systemic illness. LBP, low back pain; MRI, magnetic resonance imaging; NSAID, nonsteroidal anti-inflammatory drug; TCA, tricyclic antidepressant. Data from Chou et al [6].

European Commission Research Directorate General guidelines

In contrast to the Dutch and US guidelines, the European guidelines recommend MRI for the diagnosis of radiculopathy in patients with cLBP ($\geq$12 weeks) [2]. As noted above, however, these guidelines are confined to the management of nonspecific LBP, they make no recommendations for the treatment of radicular pain.

North American Spine Society guidelines

Radiculopathy is commonly caused by lumbar spinal stenosis [13], evidence-based guidelines for the management of this condition have been published by the NASS [9]. The key recommendations of these guidelines are summarised in Table 5.3. The guidelines emphasise the central role of MRI in the diagnosis of lumbar spine stenosis; CT myelography or CT scanning is recommended if MRI is contraindicated or inconclusive.

There is insufficient evidence to make recommendations about the benefits of pharmacological therapy with agents such as calcitonin, or nonpharmacological interventions such as physical therapy or spinal manipulation, in the management of lumbar spine stenosis. However, the guidelines note that there is fair evidence that epidural steroid injections

Principal recommendations of the NASS guidelines for the diagnosis and treatment of lumbar spinal stenosis	
Diagnosis	**Recommendation**
The diagnosis of lumbar spinal stenosis may be considered in older patients with a history of gluteal or leg symptoms exacerbated by walking or standing, which improves or resolves with sitting or bending forward. Patients whose pain is not exacerbated by walking have a low likelihood of stenosis.	Grade C
In patients with history and physical examination findings consistent with degenerative lumbar stenosis, MRI is suggested as the most appropriate noninvasive test to confirm the presence of anatomical narrowing of the spinal canal, or the presence of nerve root involvement.	Grade B
If MRI is contraindicated, CT myelography is suggested as the most appropriate test.	Grade B
If both MRI and CT myelography are contraindicated, inconclusive or inappropriate, CT is the preferred test to confirm the presence of anatomical narrowing of the spinal canal, or the presence of nerve root involvement.	Grade B
MRI or CT with axial loading is suggested as a useful adjunct to routine imaging in patients with clinical signs and symptoms of lumbar spinal stenosis, a dural sac area <110mm^2 at one or more levels and suspected central or lateral stenosis on routine unloaded MRI or CT.	Grade B
Well-defined and validated criteria for anatomical canal narrowing on MRI, CT myelography and CT should be used to improve interobserver and intraobserver reliability.	Grade B
Electromyographic paraspinal mapping is suggested to confirm the diagnosis of degenerative lumbar spinal stenosis in patients with mild or moderate symptoms and radiographic evidence of stenosis.	Grade B

Table 5.3 Principal recommendations of the NASS guidelines for the diagnosis and treatment of lumbar spinal stenosis (continues overleaf).

Principal recommendations of the NASS guidelines for the diagnosis and treatment of lumbar spinal stenosis (continued)

Medical/interventional treatment	Recommendation
Interlaminar epidural steroid injections are suggested to provide short-term (2 weeks to 6 months) symptom relief in patients with neurogenic claudication or radiculopathy. There is, however, conflicting evidence concerning long-term (21.5–24 months) efficacy.	Grade B
• Contrast-enhanced fluoroscopy is recommended to guide epidural steroid injections to improve the accuracy of medication delivery.	Grade A
A multiple injection regimen of radiographically-guided transforaminal epidural steroid injection or caudal injections is suggested to produce medium-term (3–36 months) relief of pain in patients with radiculopathy or neurogenic intermittent claudication (NIC) from lumbar spinal stenosis.	Grade C
The use of a lumbosacral corset is suggested to increase walking distance and decrease pain in patients with lumbar spinal stenosis. There is no evidence that results are sustained once the brace is removed.	Grade B
Medical/interventional treatment may be considered to provide long-term (2–10 years) improvement in patients with degenerative lumbar spinal stenosis and has been shown to improve outcomes in a large percentage of patients.	Grade C
Surgical treatment	
Decompressive surgery is suggested to improve outcomes in patients with moderate to severe symptoms of lumbar spinal stenosis:	Grade C
• Medical/interventional treatment may be considered for patients with moderate symptoms of lumbar spinal stenosis.	Grade B
• Decompression alone is suggested for patients with symptoms predominantly affecting the legs, without instability.	Grade C
• Surgical decompression may be considered in patients age ≥75 years with lumbar spinal stenosis.	Grade C
Surgical treatment may be considered to provide long-term (>4 years) improvement in patients with degenerative lumbar spinal stenosis and has been shown to improve outcomes in a large percentage of patients.	Grade C

Table 5.3 Principal recommendations of the NASS guidelines for the diagnosis and treatment of lumbar spinal stenosis (continued). Grade A recommendations, good evidence (consistent results from high-quality randomised controlled trials) to support an intervention; Grade B recommendations, fair evidence to support an intervention; Grade C recommendations, poor-quality evidence to support an intervention. Grade A recommendations indicate that an intervention is 'recommended', whereas Grade B recommendations indicate that the intervention is 'suggested' and Grade C recommendations indicate that the intervention 'may be considered'. Data from the North American Spine Society [9].

can provide short-term (up to 6 months) pain relief, although the long-term benefits of such treatment are less clear. There is strong evidence from high-quality clinical trials to support the use of contrast-enhanced fluoroscopy to guide epidural steroid injections.

The NASS guidelines suggest that decompressive surgery should be used in patients with moderate to severe symptoms, and there is limited evidence to suggest that such treatment can provide long-term (>4 years) improvement in patients with degenerative lumbar spinal stenosis.

American Society of Interventional Pain Physicians guidelines

The American Society of Interventional Pain Physicians (ASIPP) has published evidence-based guidelines for the management of patients with chronic spinal pain, including radicular pain [14]. In contrast to most other guidelines, these are intended for use by pain specialists. The principal recommendations in these guidelines that relate to the management of radiculopathy are:

- There is moderate evidence to support the use of transforaminal epidural injections or selective nerve root blockade in the preoperative evaluation of patients in whom imaging provides negative or inconclusive results.
- In patients with chronic low back and radicular pain, there is strong evidence that caudal epidural steroid injections provide short-term pain relief and moderate evidence for long-term benefit.
- In patients with lumbar radiculopathy, there is strong evidence that interlaminar epidural steroid injections provide effective short-term pain relief and limited evidence for long-term relief; by contrast, there is only moderate evidence that such procedures are beneficial in patients with cervical radiculopathy.

References

1   van Tulder M, Becker A, Bekkering T, et al. European guidelines for the management of acute nonspecific low back pain in primary care. *Eur Spine J.* 2006;15:S169-191.
2   Airaksinen O, Brox JI, Cedraschi C, et al. European guidelines for the management of chronic nonspecific low back pain. *Eur Spine J.* 2006;15:S192-300.
3   Waddell G, McIntosh A, Hutchinson A, Feder G, Lewis M. Low Back Pain Evidence Review London: Royal College of General Practitioners. 1999. Available at: www.chiro.org/LINKS/GUIDELINES/FULL/Royal_College/index.html. Accessed September 25, 2012.
4   National Institute for Health and Clinical Excellence. Clinical Guideline 88: Low Back Pain. Available at: www.nice.org.uk/CG88fullguideline. Accessed September 25, 2012.
5   Mens JMA, Chavannes AW, Koes BW, et al. NHG-Standaard Lumbosacraal radiculair syndroom (in Dutch). *Huisarts Wet.* 2005;48:178-178.

6   Chou R, Qaseem A, Snow V, et al. Diagnosis and treatment of low back pain: a joint clinical practice guideline from the American College of Physicians and the American Pain Society. *Ann Intern Med.* 2007;147:478-491.

7   Chou R, Huffman LH. Nonpharmacologic therapies for acute and chronic low back pain: a review of the evidence for an American Pain Society/American College of Physicians clinical practice guideline. *Ann Intern Med.* 2007;147:492-504.

8   Chou R, Huffman LH. Medications for acute and chronic low back pain: a review of the evidence for an American Pain Society/American College of Physicians clinical practice guideline. *Ann Intern Med.* 2007;147:505-514.

9   North American Spine Society. Evidence-based clinical guidelines for multidisciplinary spine care. Available at: www.spine.org/Pages/PracticePolicy/ClinicalCare/ClinicalGuidelines/Default.aspx. Accessed September 25, 2012.

10 Koes BW, van Tulder MW, Ostelo R, Kim Burton A, Waddell G. Clinical guidelines for the management of low back pain in primary care: an international comparison. *Spine.* 2001;26:2504-2513.

11 Koes BW, van Tulder MW, Peul WC. Diagnosis and treatment of sciatica. *BMJ.* 2007;334:1313-1317.

12 Modic MT, Obuchowski NA, Ross JS, et al. Acute low back pain and radiculopathy: MR imaging findings and their prognostic role and effect on outcome. *Radiology.* 2005;237:597-604.

13 Binder DK, Schmidt MH, Weinstein PR. Lumbar spinal stenosis. *Semin Neurol.* 2002;22:157-166.

14 Boswell MV, Trescot AM, Datta S, et al. Interventional techniques: evidence-based practice guidelines in the management of chronic spinal pain. *Pain Physician.* 2007;10:7-111.

Development of this book was supported by funding from Pfizer

Chapter 6

Physical and psychological treatments

Kika Konstantinou and Joanne L. Jordan

Treatment options for radiculopathy

In this chapter the current evidence on the effectiveness of conservative, non-invasive, non-pharmacological treatment options for the conditions of lumbar and cervical radicular pain are summarised. These include active physiotherapy interventions in the form of exercises, passive physiotherapy interventions such as manual therapy, traction, acupuncture, heat and cold applications, massage, electrotherapy interventions such as the use of transcutaneous electrical nerve stimulation (TENS) units, collars, spinal braces and supports, rest, psychological interventions such as cognitive-behavioural therapy (CBT) or behavioural therapy and interventions to address occupational barriers to recovery. Presented in this chapter is a summary of the results from the most recent systematic and other reviews evaluating the evidence for the effectiveness of the aforementioned treatment options [1–9]; randomised controlled trials (RCTs) [10–18] that have been published after the most recent systematic review on the subject have also been included. The most recent and comprehensive systematic review by Lewis et al [4] informs the majority of recommendations on conservative treatments for radicular pain due to disc herniation (Table 6.1) [19].

F. Laroche and S. Perrot (eds.), *Managing Sciatica and Radicular Pain in Primary Care Practice*, DOI: 10.1007/978-1-907673-56-6_6, © Springer Healthcare 2013

Summary of studies on sciatica

Study	Type of research	Inclusion criteria	Intervention	Comparison
Lewis 2011 [4]	Systematic review Search date: December 2009	Sciatica	Traction	Inactive control
				Usual care
				Exercise therapy
				Passive physiotherapy
				Exercise alone (versus exercise + traction)
				Activity restriction alone (versus activity restriction + traction)
				All comparisons
			Spinal manipulation	Inactive control (sham manipulation; soft tissue pressing without any rapid thrust)
				All comparisons
			Acupuncture	Inactive control (sham acupuncture; non-acupuncture points or needling not penetrating the skin)
			Alternative therapy (including acupuncture)	Inactive control
				Usual care
				Activity restriction
				Education/advice
			Active physiotherapy/ exercise therapy	All comparisons
				Inactive control
			Exercise therapy	Usual care
				Activity restriction
			Exercise + passive physiotherapy	Activity restriction

Table 6.1 Summary of studies on sciatica (continues overleaf).

Outcome	Conclusion	Length of follow up	Evidence/quality
All outcomes	No difference	Short- to medium-term	1 or 2 moderate quality RCTs
All outcomes	No difference	Short- to medium-term	2 moderate and 1 poor quality RCTs
Pain	Positive	Short-term	1 moderate RCT
Global effect	No difference		
Condition-specific outcome			
Adverse effect	Negative		
All outcomes	No difference	Medium-term	Mixed treatment comparison
Global effect	No difference Positive		1 good RCT
All outcomes	No difference	Medium-term	Mixed treatment comparison
Pain	Positive	Short-term	1 moderate RCT
Pain	Positive	Medium-term	Mixed treatment comparison
All outcomes	No difference	Medium-term	Mixed treatment comparison
Pain	Positive	Short-term	1 moderate crossover RCT
Condition-specific function	Negative	Short-term	1 good RCT
Global effect	Positive	Long-term	
Other outcomes	No difference	Other time points	
Global effect	No difference	Short-term	1 poor RCT
Function	Positive	Short-term	1 moderate RCT

Summary of studies on sciatica (continued)

Study	Type of research	Inclusion criteria	Intervention	Comparison
			Passive physiotherapy (TENS)	Inactive control
			Activity restriction	Advice to stay active
				Usual care
Ernst & Lee 2010 [5]	Overview of SRs Search date: 2000 to 2010 (date not reported)	All rheumatological conditions (including one SR of people with sciatica)	Acupuncture	Not known
Albert & Manniche 2012 [11]	RCT 181 patients	Severe sciatica (leg pain at least to knee of >3 on 1–10 point scale lasting 2 weeks to 1 year)	Active, symptom-guided exercise (based on McKenzie principles)	'Sham' exercises (optional low-dose not back-related)
Konstantinovic 2010 [10]	RCT 546 patients	Acute low back pain with radiculopathy (<4 weeks)	Low-level laser therapy (LLLT) + nimesulide (200mg/day)	Sham LLLT + nimesulide Nimesulide alone

Table 6.1 Summary of studies on sciatica (continued). The explanations of the conclusions are as follows: positive, statistically significant difference in outcome between groups in favour of the intervention; negative, statistically significant difference in outcome between groups in favour of the comparison group; no difference, the differences in outcome between groups is not statistically significant; inconsistent, the results vary between trials/studies; insufficient

Physiotherapy treatment options

The evidence on non-pharmacological, non-surgical treatments described in the following section refers to disc-related lumbar radicular symptoms.

Exercise therapy for disc related sciatica

Active physiotherapy or exercise therapy is generally recommended for patients with lumbar radicular pain that fails to improve naturally

Outcome	Conclusion	Length of follow up	Evidence/quality
Pain	Positive	Short-term	1 poor crossover RCT
Global effect			
Condition-specific outcomes	Negative	Short-term	2 moderate RCTs
Other outcomes	No difference	Short- and medium-term	
Pain	Negative	Medium-term	Mixed treatment comparison
Not known	Positive	Not known	1 poor SR of 6 mostly poor quality studies
Leg pain	No difference	Short- and medium-term	High quality*
Global effect	Positive		
Pain intensity	Positive (Positive [sham vs nimesulide])	Short-term	High quality*
Function/ disability	Positive (Positive [sham vs nimesulide])		

evidence, too few studies were found comparing these interventions to judge their effectiveness. The length of the follow up are as follows: short-term, <6 weeks; medium-term, ≥6 weeks to 6 months; long-term, >6 months. RCT, randomised controlled trials; SRs, systematic reviews; TENS, transcutaneous electrical nerve stimulation. *Quality assessed using Cochrane Risk of Bias Tool. Data from Higgins & Green [19].

in a short period of time. Exercise programmes may consist of lumbar strengthening and/or stretching exercises, general functional exercises, specific strengthening spinal exercises such as lumbar stabilisation exercises or extension-orientated exercises (McKenzie approach). Lumbar stabilisation exercises (also referred to as 'core stability') refer to these exercises that target the abdominal, low back and pelvic area muscles. The assumption is that weakness in those muscles may contribute to back pain and its persistence. A specific exercise programme is tailored to the patient and progression of exercises is made accordingly. Figure 6.1 provides simple examples of these stability exercises. The McKenzie method explores the response of pain in the back or radiating from the back to directional mechanical forces, predominately repeated spinal movements [20,21]. Pain that tends to improve in terms of location and severity and eventually ceases due to certain positions and movements of the spine is attributed to the centralisation phenomenon. Centralisation describes the relocation of pain from a distal site proximally toward the midline. The response to repeated movements is used in clinical practice as an assessment and treatment method. It is advisable that patients receive treatment utilising this approach by qualified practitioners with relevant training in this method.

Studies comparing exercise therapy to no treatment or alternative interventions show that there is no strong evidence for the effectiveness of exercise for any outcomes (such as pain, function, perceived improvement or recurrences) over other interventions [4]. The most comprehensive systematic review by Lewis et al reported that there is some evidence to suggest that active exercises produce better pain improvements in the short term and better global improvements in the long term [4]. However, their analysis did not find any statistical significance for the use of active exercises in improving outcomes in disc-related sciatica. Individual RCTs in this review provide limited evidence of positive results [22,23]. One trial, comparing no treatment with lumbar stabilisation exercise, reported short-term improvements in pain [18]. One good quality RCT supported the use of physiotherapy/exercises in addition to general practitioner care for patients with severe sciatica for global improvement [23]. A more recent study by Albert et al provides evidence for the effectiveness of exercise in general and symptom-guided exercises in particular (based on the McKenzie principles and with the addition of spinal stabilising exercises) for severe sciatica for outcomes of global improvement, long-term sick leave from employment, neurological deficits and patient satisfaction compared to sham exercises (these were described as non-related to the spine and were optional) [11].

Spine strengthening exercises

A

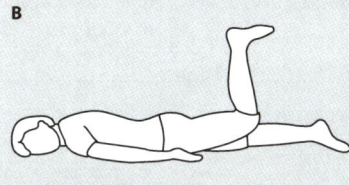

Stomach tone ('transverse tummy')
The patient should lay down on their front head facing over one shoulder. They should pull in their stomach muscles, while maintaining breathing, centred around the navel and hold for 5 seconds, this should be repeated three times. The exercise should build up to 10 seconds and repeat during the day, for example while walking or standing

B

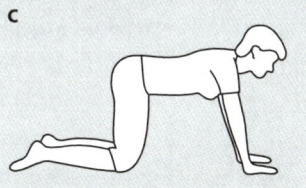

Buttock tone (gluteals)
Laying face down on the floor the patient should bend one leg up behind them, then lift their bent knee just off the floor. The patient should hold for 8 seconds if possible and repeat five times on each side

C

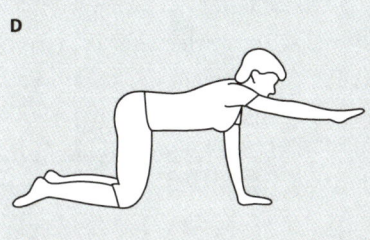

Deep stomach muscle tone
The patient should kneel on all fours with a small curve in the lower back, the stomach should be completely relaxed. Pull the lower part of the stomach upwards so that the back is lifted (without arching) away from the floor

D

Back stabiliser
The patient should kneel on all fours with their back straight and tighten their stomach. Keeping the back in this position, raise one arm in front and hold for 10 seconds. The pelvis should be kept level and the body should not rotate. This should be repeated for 10 times each side. As the patient progresses they can try to lift one leg behind them instead of their arm

Figure 6.1 Spine strengthening exercises. These exercises should be recommended with caution and during supervision with a healthcare professional. Reproduced with permission from Arthritis Research UK.

Although the collective evidence from systematic reviews is insufficient to support the effectiveness of active exercises, evidence from individual RCTs suggests that exercises in disc-related sciatica may be effective and should be considered as a treatment option with usual general practitioner care for patients that do not seem to improve over time, before referral to secondary care services [11,18,23].

Manual therapy

Manual therapy is the collective term for describing joint mobilisation and manipulation techniques. Joint mobilisation is defined as passive oscillatory movements and joint manipulation is defined as small amplitude thrust or stretch applied at high speed at the limit of the available range of movement. Physiotherapists, osteopaths and chiropractors may use these techniques in treating low back pain (LBP) with or without radicular pain.

Santilli et al [24] reported that manipulation was superior to sham manipulation (soft tissue pressing without any rapid thrust) for medium-term effects (between 6 to 12 months) for global improvement. However, the analysis of this study by Lewis et al did not provide any evidence that manipulation/mobilisation interventions are beneficial for sciatica [4].

Overall there is limited evidence that manipulation/mobilisation may be effective in sciatica although further research may change the strength of this evidence. Nonspecific LBP guidelines recommend the use of manipulation/mobilisation [25–27]. This evidence comes from studies that normally have mixed populations (nonspecific LBP and sciatica) where it is not possible to separately report outcomes for patients with sciatica. Considering the overall evidence, it is reasonable to suggest that the use of manipulation/mobilisation may be based on patient and clinician preference until further research evidence is available regarding its effectiveness. The popularity of these approaches may also depend on cultural preferences and expectations and thus vary between countries and practitioners.

Traction

The systematic review by Lewis et al reported that there was no important difference between traction and inactive comparison or alternative comparison [4]. None of the studies included was of good quality and none reported long-term outcomes. Two other systematic reviews that included mixed populations of patients with and without radicular pain reached the same conclusion [1,2]. Collectively, these reviews do not recommend the use of traction in sciatica.

Acupuncture

The systematic review by Lewis et al [4] assessed the effectiveness of acupuncture compared with sham acupuncture (non-acupuncture points or needling not penetrating the skin) or other alternative treatments for sciatica. Overall, the authors concluded that true acupuncture may be more effective than sham acupuncture for pain relief in the short term [4], suggesting that acupuncture may be beneficial for sciatica.

Generally, the evidence for acupuncture in lumbar radiculopathy is very sparse and of low quality [2,4,5] and further high-quality research is needed to evaluate the benefit of acupuncture compared with sham acupuncture or current usual care. In clinical practice, however, acupuncture is used for symptomatic pain relief and its use has been recommended for the treatment of LBP [27,28]. It is reasonable to suggest that the use of acupuncture is based on patient and clinician preference until further research evidence is available regarding its effectiveness. Cultural mores may also influence the use of acupuncture.

Passive physiotherapy interventions
Heat, ice and massage

Heat and cold applications (hot/cold packs) are commonly used by people with LBP and at times by health professionals. A Cochrane review [29] found heat therapy to be better than placebo in the short term for pain relief and functional status for acute LBP. However, the evidence on cold applications is very limited and of poor quality and no conclusions could be made [29]. Massage also may be used for people with LBP but there is conflicting evidence regarding its effectiveness [26].

There are no studies investigating the effect of these measures in patients with sciatica and, there are therefore no specific recommendations in this setting [2,4]. However, patients with sciatica may be advised to try heat or cold applications to the lower back area for symptomatic pain relief at home if they feel these measures provide any benefit, in addition to any other conservative treatment they receive. Adverse effects for using such measures are considered minimal and a trial use may be reasonable depending on individual patient preferences.

Electrotherapy

Lewis et al [4] identified one poor quality crossover RCT that compared TENS or percutaneous electrical nerve stimulation (PENS) to inactive control for patients with both radicular and referred pain. This study reported a significant short-term improvement in pain for the interventions but, based on the quality of this evidence, TENS/PENS are not recommended as a treatment for sciatica due to disc prolapse.

One good quality RCT investigated the effects (short-term) of low-level laser therapy for patients with acute, disc-related sciatica (short duration of symptoms) [10]. After 3 weeks of treatment they concluded that this intervention, as an additional therapy to medication, resulted in significant improvements in all outcomes measured (including pain intensity, lumbar movement and quality of life), which were over and above a placebo effect. However, the intervention was intensive, 15 minutes of treatment, every day for 3 weeks and patients were hospitalised. Although the results appear promising in the short term, more evidence will be required before a recommendation is made for the use of such intensive laser therapy in disc-related sciatica.

Back braces or supports

Lumbar supports may be flexible or rigid and they are sometimes used or favoured by people with LBP. Overall, there is insufficient review evidence on the effectiveness of lumbar supports for back pain [25], and no evidence at all in relation to sciatica, consequently no recommendations related to this setting can be made [2,4].

Bed rest and inactivity

The systematic review by Lewis et al [4] reports that rest and inactivity has a negative effect on outcomes for disc-related sciatica although, overall, the difference between advice to stay active and rest is small. However, it is reasonable to suggest that it is preferable that patients with sciatica remain as active as possible as prolonged rest and avoidance of activities would lead to deconditioning and possible delay in improvement. This is in line with moderate evidence from studies on LBP suggesting that advice to remain active leads to better outcome compared with advice to rest [30].

Psychological therapies

There are a number of studies on psychological therapies (ie, psychotherapy, CBT, behavioural therapy) for treating nonspecific LBP [31,32].

CBT is based on the idea that thoughts cause feelings and behaviours, not external stressors, such as people, situations and events. This type of psychotherapy aims to change the way patients think, to challenge their beliefs about their pain and condition and therefore to change their behaviour and hopefully reduce disability and improve quality of life. Another type of psychotherapy is behavioural therapy, or behavioural modification. This technique is based on the premise that specific, observable, maladaptive, badly adjusted or self-destructing behaviours can be modified by learning new, more appropriate behaviours to replace them. The focus in this context is treatment for changing and modifying pain behaviour.

No recommendations can be made for the use of psychological therapies in the treatment of sciatica as no information from RCTs could be found. The treating clinician and the patient may consider psychological therapies when other appropriate treatments have failed or when the patient feels distressed by the symptoms and is unable to cope with the subsequent compromise of quality of life.

Summary of treatment options for disc-related sciatica
- There is evidence to suggest that activity restriction and traction should not be recommended in sciatica due to disc herniation.
- There is evidence from two high quality RCTs that exercise (active physiotherapy) is effective.
- There is limited evidence that manual therapy (manipulation) may be effective.

- There is limited and indirect evidence that acupuncture may be effective.
- There is evidence from one RCT that low-level laser therapy may be effective in the short-term when added to medication although treatment was very intensive and may not be applicable in most settings.

Targeted approaches

The use of combinations of the strategies already discussed in this chapter is central to targeted treatment approaches, which are designed to tailor treatment to individual patients depending on their presenting symptoms or patient subgroups: the ultimate goal of such approaches is to improve patient outcomes and increase cost efficiency. One study demonstrated that the subgrouping of LBP patients as; at low, medium or high risk of poor prognosis and then targeting interventions appropriate to each subgroup seems to work well overall in primary care as compared to usual care [33]. However, the results of this study are applicable to nonspecific LBP and it is not presently known whether this approach is directly applicable to specific presentations such as disc related sciatica or spinal stenosis, although such an approach may be considered as an adjunct to clinical judgement. Screening and stratification may also be useful when addressing occupational risk factors, although again the evidence comes from studies on patients with nonspecific LBP.

Treatment options for cervical radicular pain

Two systematic reviews [6,7] and six RCTs not included in these reviews [12–17] have investigated the effectiveness of non-pharmacological, non-surgical interventions for cervical radicular pain (Table 6.2) [19].

The systematic review by Gross et al [6] included studies of populations with neck pain with or without radiculopathy. However, the authors reported there was insufficient evidence for the effectiveness of manual therapy specifically for those patients with symptoms of radiculopathy. Similarly, another systematic review [7] also reported insufficient evidence for the effectiveness of exercises (physiotherapy), manual therapy, collars, traction, electrotherapy (eg, TENS) for cervical radiculopathy.

Traction

There is conflicting evidence for the short-term effects of traction added to manual therapy and exercises from two small, moderate-quality RCTs [15,16]. In addition, no difference in medium-term outcomes was noted with the addition of traction to conventional rehabilitation including manual therapy in one of these moderate-quality RCTs [16].

Cervical collar

Evidence from one low quality RCT shows that long-term outcomes for patients with at least 3 months' duration of symptoms are equal for physiotherapy and collar [12]. One moderate-quality RCT showed that the short-term effect for patients with symptom durations of less than 1 month is the same for physiotherapy and exercises or the use of a collar, both interventions gave additional reduction in pain over the control group ('wait and see' policy) [15]. There were no differences between all interventions at 6 months.

Manual therapy

There is limited evidence from one small, moderate-quality RCT that a combination of manual therapy and exercises has better short-term effects compared with each modality alone [14].

Laser therapy

There is evidence from one small, high-quality RCT that laser treatment has better short-term effects on arm pain and functional disability compared with sham laser (laser unit inactive) for acute radicular symptoms [17]. However, there was no statistical difference in neck pain between the active and sham laser treatment groups. The potential benefits of laser therapy need to be assessed in larger RCTs, as this sample was highly selected (out of 285 assessed for eligibility, 200 did not meet inclusion criteria). The intervention was intensive, with 15 minutes of treatment, every day for 3 weeks, during which time the patients were hospitalised.

Summary of studies of cervical radiculopathy

Study	Type of research	Inclusion criteria	Intervention	Comparison
Gross et al 2010 [6]	Systematic review Search date: July 2009	Neck pain with or without radiculopathy	Manipulation or mobilisation	Any comparison
Bono et al 2011 [7]	Evidence-based clinical guidelines Search date: May 2009	Cervical radiculopathy caused by degenerative disorders	Physical therapy/ exercise Manipulation/ chiropractic therapy Bracing, traction, electrical stimulation, acupuncture, TENS	Any comparison
Persson et al 1997 [12]	RCT 81 patients	Cervicobrachial pain with clinical and radiological confirmed nerve root compression (>3 months duration)	Physiotherapy (including individualised exercises, TENs, heat or cold, massage, manual therapy, relaxation)	Cervical collar (Also included a group receiving surgery)
Ragonese 2009 [13]	RCT 30 patients	Cervical radiculopathy (unknown duration)	Manual therapy and exercise programme (standardised)	Manual therapy or exercise programme alone
Kuijper et al 2009 [14]	RCT 205 patients	Cervical radiculopathy (<1 month duration)	Physiotherapy and home exercises Cervical collar and rest	Continued normal activities (wait and see policy)
Young et al 2009 [15]	RCT 81 patients	Cervical radiculopathy (52% <3 months' duration)	Manual therapy, exercise and intermittent cervical traction	Manual therapy, exercise and sham traction/exercises (non-related to the spine and are optional)
Jellad et al 2009 [16]	RCT 39 patients	Cervical radiculopathy (<3 months' duration)	Conventional rehabilitation including either manual or intermittent traction	Conventional rehabilitation alone
Konstantinovic 2010 [17]	RCT 60 patients	Acute neck pain with radiculopathy (<4 weeks duration)	Low-level laser therapy	Sham low-level laser therapy (laser unit inactive)

Table 6.2 Summary of studies of cervical radiculopathy. The explanations of the conclusions are as follows: positive, statistically significant difference in outcome between groups in favour of the intervention; negative, statistically significant difference in outcome between groups in favour of the comparison group; no difference, the differences in outcome between groups is not statistically significant; inconsistent, the results vary between trials/studies; insufficient

Outcome	Conclusion	Length of follow up	Evidence/quality
Any outcome	Insufficient evidence for those with radiculopathy	N/A	Unknown
Any outcome	Insufficient evidence	N/A	Unknown
	Insufficient evidence – suggests negative effect		
	Insufficient evidence – suggests positive effect		
Pain	No difference	Short- and long-term	Low quality
Function (overall scores)	Positive	Short-term	
	No difference	Long-term	
Pain function (NDI)	Positive	Post intervention	Moderate quality
Mean weekly change in arm and neck pain	Positive	Short-term	Moderate quality
Mean weekly change in function (NDI)	No difference		
Mean weekly change in arm and neck pain and function (NDI)	Positive		
Pain function (NDI)	No difference	Short-term	Moderate quality
Cervical and radicular pain	Positive	Post-intervention	Moderate quality
Function/disability			
	No difference	Medium-term	
Arm pain	Positive	Short-term	High quality
Function/disability			
Neck pain	No difference		

evidence, too few studies were found comparing these interventions to judge their effectiveness. The length of the follow up are as follows: short-term, <6 weeks; medium-term, >6 weeks to 6 months; long-term, >6 months. NDI, Neck Disability Index; RCT, randomised controlled trials; TENS, transcutaneous electrical nerve stimulation. *Quality assessed using Cochrane Risk of Bias Tool. Data from Higgins & Green [19].

> *Summary of treatment options for cervical radicular pain*
> - There is limited evidence for the effectiveness of physiotherapy (exercises) and manual therapy.
> - There is conflicting evidence for the effectiveness of traction and low to moderate evidence that physiotherapy and exercises provide similar short-term results compared to collars.
> - Limited evidence supports the use of intensive laser treatment for short duration symptoms and short-term effects.

Treatment options for lumbar spinal stenosis

Radicular pain may also be caused by spinal stenosis (either central or lateral). There are two systematic reviews on the effectiveness of conservative interventions for lumbar spinal stenosis [8,9] and one recently published RCT [18] not included in these reviews (Table 6.3) [19].

Summary table for lumbar spinal stenosis

Study	Type of research	Inclusion criteria	Intervention	Comparison
Reiman et al 2009 [8]	Systematic review Search date: October 2007	Lumbar spinal stenosis	Manual therapy (as part of physiotherapy package	Physiotherapy package without manual therapy
Watters et al 2008 [9]	Evidence-based clinical guidelines	Lumbar spinal stenosis	Lumbosacral corset	Unknown
	Search date: April 2006		Physical therapy/exercise	Any comparison
			Manipulation/chiropractic therapy	
			Traction, electrical stimulation, acupuncture, TENS	
Goren et al 2010 [18]	RCT 45 patients	Lumbar spinal stenosis (MRI-proven; 68% had lumbar spinal stenosis for >1 year)	Exercise + ultrasound	No treatment or exercise
			Exercise + sham ultrasound	
			Exercise + ultrasound	Exercise + sham ultrasound

Table 6.3 Summary table for lumbar spinal stenosis. The explanations of the conclusions are as follows: positive is a statistically significant difference in outcome between groups in favour of the intervention; negative is a statistically significant difference in outcome between groups in favour of the comparison group; no difference, the differences in outcome between groups is not statistically significant; inconsistent means that the results vary between trials/studies; insufficient

The review by Reiman et al concluded that physiotherapy with the addition of manual therapy techniques have a positive short- and long-term outcome compared with physiotherapy packages without manual therapy in patients with lumbar spinal stenosis [8].

However, another systematic review concluded that there was insufficient evidence for the use of physical therapy, including exercises, manual therapy, traction and other passive interventions such as acupuncture and TENS, for all comparisons and all outcomes in this setting [9]. Short-term positive evidence from poor-quality studies for the use of lumbosacral corsets for pain and walking distance outcomes were cited in this review but no information regarding the comparison interventions was provided.

One small RCT of moderate quality evaluated the effect of adding ultrasound (US) to active exercise compared with no exercise and showed that pain and disability were reduced in the exercise groups irrespective of the addition of active or placebo US, suggesting that the results

Outcome	Conclusion	Length of follow up	Evidence/quality
Global effect	Positive	Short- and long-term	1 RCT and consistent findings from several observational studies (Level 2 van Tulder criteria [28])
Pain	Positive	Short-term	Poor quality studies
Walking distance			
Any outcome	Insufficient evidence	N/A	
	Insufficient evidence		
	Insufficient evidence		
Leg pain	Positive	Short-term	Moderate quality
Function/disability			
Leg pain	No difference		
Function/disability			

evidence means that too few studies were found comparing these interventions to judge their effectiveness. The length of the follow up are as follows: short-term, <6 weeks; medium-term, >6 weeks to 6 months; long-term, >6 months. MRI, magnetic resonance imaging; RCT, randomised controlled trials; TENS, transcutaneous electrical nerve stimulation. *Quality assessed using Cochrane Risk of Bias Tool. Data from Higgins & Green [19].

are due to the exercises compared with an inactive treatment and not the addition of the US [18].

There is limited evidence for the effectiveness of physiotherapy (exercises) and manual therapy in patients with spinal stenosis. It would be reasonable to recommend a course of physiotherapy, including exercises and manual therapy, at the discretion of the therapist and according to patient preference, when a patient does not present with severe clinical symptoms of spinal stenosis and for whom surgical interventions are not as yet appropriate. Passive treatments such as electrotherapy, traction and corsets are not recommended.

Maintaining improvements and avoiding recurrence

Following a successful outcome with any of the treatments discussed in this chapter, the doctor or physiotherapist will advise his/her patient on strategies to reduce the chances of recurrence of the problem. Although there is no evidence on strategies which would minimise recurrences of disc-related sciatica and symptoms due to stenosis, it is reasonable to suggest that healthy, active lifestyles and regular physical activity are likely to be beneficial in reducing the odds of recurrence and keep symptoms at bay.

References

1   Luijsterburg PAJ, Verhagen AP, Ostelo R, et al. Effectiveness of conservative treatments for the lumbosacral radicular syndrome: a systematic review. *Eur Spine J.* 2007;16:881-899.
2   Jordan J, Konstantinou K, O'Dowd J. Herniated lumbar disc. *Clin Evid (Online).* 2011. pii:1118.
3   Hahne AJ, Ford JJ, McMeeken JM. Conservative management of lumbar disc herniation with associated radiculopathy: a systematic review. *Spine.* 2010;35:E488-E504.
4   Lewis R, Wiliams N, Matar HE, et al. The clinical effectiveness and cost-effectiveness of management strategies for sciatica: systematic review and economic model. *Health Technol Assess.* 2011;15:1-578.
5   Ernst E, Lee MS. Acupuncture for rheumatic conditions: an overview of systematic reviews. *Rheumatology.* 2010;49:1957-1961.
6   Gross A, Miller J, D'Sylva J, et al. Manipulation or mobilisation for neck pain. *Cochrane Database Syst Rev.* 2010;1:CD004249.
7   Bono CM, Ghiselli G, Gilbert TJ, et al. An evidence-based clinical guideline for the diagnosis and treatment of cervical radiculopathy from degenerative disorders. *Spine J.* 2011;11:64-72.
8   Reiman MP, Harris JY, Cleland JA. Manual therapy interventions for patients with lumbar spinal stenosis: a systematic review. *NZJ Physiother.* 2009;37:17-28.
9   Watters WC, Baisden J, Gilbert TJ, et al. Degenerative lumbar spinal stenosis: an evidence-based clinical guideline for the diagnosis and treatment of degenerative lumbar spinal stenosis. *Spine J.* 2008;8:305-310.
10 Konstantinovic LM, Kanjuh ZM, Milovanovic AN, et al. Acute low back pain with radiculopathy: a double-blind, randomized, placebo-controlled study. *Photomed Laser Surg.* 2010;28:553-560.
11 Albert HB, Manniche C. The efficacy of systematic active conservative treatment for patients with severe sciatica. *Spine.* 2012;37:531-542.

12 Persson LC, Carlsson C-A, Carlsson JY. Long-lasting cervical radicular pain managed with surgery, physiotherapy, or a cervical collar: a prospective, randomized study. *Spine*. 1997;22:751-758.

13 Ragonese J. A randomized trial comparing manual physical therapy to therapeutic exercises, to a combination of therapies, for the treatment of cervical radiculopathy. *Orthopaedic Pract*. 2009;21:71-76.

14 Kuijper B, Tans JTJ, Beelen A, Nollet F, de Visser M. Cervical collar or physiotherapy versus wait and see policy for recent onset cervical radiculopathy: randomized trial. *BMJ*. 2009;339:b3883.

15 Young IA, Michener LA, Cleland JA, Aguilera AJ, Snyder AR. Manual therapy, exercise and traction for patients with cervical radiculopathy: a randomized clinical trial. *Physical Ther*. 2009;89:632-642.

16 Jellad A, Ben Salah Z, Boudokhane S, Migaou H, Bahri I, Rejeb N. The value of intermittent cervical traction in recent cervical radiculopathy. *Ann Phys Rehabil Med*. 2009;52:638-652.

17 Konstantinovic LM, Cutovic MR, Milovanovic AN, et al. Low-level laser therapy for acute neck pain with radiculopathy: a double-blind placebo-controlled randomized study. 2010;11:1169-1178.

18 Goren A, Yildiz N, Topuz O, Findikoglu G, Ardic F. Efficacy of exercise and ultrasound in patients with lumbar spinal stenosis: a prospective randomised trial. *Clin Rehab*. 2010;24:623-631.

19 Higgins JPT, Green S, eds. *Cochrane Handbook for Systematic Reviews of Interventions. Version 5.1.0* [updated March 2011]. The Cochrane Collaboration, 2011. Available at: www.cochrane-handbook.org. Accessed September 4, 2012.

20 McKenzie RA, May S. *The Cervical and Thoracic Spine: Mechanical Diagnosis and Therapy*. 2nd edn. Waikanae: Spinal Publications New Zealand; 2006.

21 McKenzie RA, May S. *The Lumbar Spine: Mechanical Diagnosis and Therapy*. Waikanae: Spinal Publications New Zealand; 2003.

22 Bakhtiary AH, Safavi-Farokhi Z, Rezasoltani A. Lumbar stabilizing exercises improve activities of daily living in patients with lumbar disc herniation. *J Back Musculoskel Rehab*. 2005;18:55-60.

23 Luijsterburg PA, Verhagen AP, Ostelo RW, et al. Physical therapy plus general practitioners' care versus general practitioners' care alone for sciatica: a randomised clinical trial with a 12 month follow-up. *Eur Spine J*. 2008;17:509-517.

24 Santilli V, Beghi E, Finucci S. Chiropractic manipulation in the treatment of acute back pain and sciatica with disc protrusion: a randomized double-blind clinical trial of active and simulated spinal manipulations. *Spine J*. 2006;6:131-137.

25 Chou R, Huffman LH. Nonpharmacologic therapies for acute and chronic low-back pain: a review of the evidence for and American Pain Society/American College of Physicians clinical practice guideline. *Annals Int Med*. 2007a;147:492-504.

26 Chou R, Qaseem A, Snow V, et al. Diagnosis and treatment of low back pain: a joint clinical practice guideline from the American College of Physicians and the American Pain Society. *Annals Int Med*. 2007b;147:478-491.

27 Savigny P, Kuntze S, Watson P, et al. low back pain: early management of persistent non-specific low back pain. London: National Institute of Clinical Evidence, 2009. Available at: www.nice.org.uk/CG88. Accessed September 4, 2012; page updated July 18, 2012.

28 van Tulder MW, Cherkin D, Berman B, Lao L, Koes BW. Acupuncture for low back pain. *Cochrane Database Syst Rev*. 1999;2:CD001351.

29 French SD, Cameron M, Walker BF, Reggars JW, Esterman AJ. Superficial heat or cold for low back pain. *Cochrane Database Syst Rev*. 2006;1:CD004750.

30 Dahm KT, Brurberg KG, Jamtvedt G, Hagen KB. Advice to rest in bed versus advice to stay active for acute low-back pain and sciatica. *Cochrane Database Syst Rev*. 2010:6:CD007612.

31 Hoffman BM, Papas RK, Chatkoff DK, Kerns RD. Meta-analysis of psychological interventions for chronic low back pain. *Health Psychol*. 2007;26:1-9.

32 Henschke N, Ostelo RWJG, van Tulder MW, et al. Behavioural treatment for chronic low-back pain. *Cochrane Database Syst Rev*. 2010;7:CD002014.

33 Hill JC, Whitehurst DGT, Lewis M, et al. Comparison of stratified primary care management for low back pain with current best practice (STartBack): a randomised controlled trial. *Lancet*. 2011;378:1560-1571.

Development of this book was supported by funding from Pfizer

Chapter 7

What are the options for the surgical treatment of radiculopathy?

Brad Williamson

Principles of surgery in patients with radiculopathy

This chapter describes the surgical options for the management of both cervical and lumbar radiculopathy. As described in Chapter 5, conservative measures form the mainstay of treatment for sciatica and such treatment will produce effective pain relief within a few weeks in most patients [1–3]. However, in approximately 10–30% of patients, pain may persist [1–4], and these patients may require surgery to attain effective pain relief. In other cases, urgent surgery is mandatory; for example, when motor deficit or cauda equina syndrome develops.

Most spinal surgery is elective, therefore the decision to operate requires consideration of the relative benefits, risks and burdens of surgery to the individual patient [5,6]. For this reason, a shared decision-making approach is appropriate, in which the patient is given clear information about the relative benefits and risks of surgery, in order to allow him or her to make an informed choice [5–7]. In patients with radiculopathy due to a prolapsed lumbar disc, an important consideration is that the benefits of surgery appear to diminish over time [5,6], that is to say there is a relative benefit in terms of a rapid relief of sciatica, but the long-term outcome is similar in those treated operatively and non-operatively. In the lumbar spine, surgery has been shown to be highly effective for radicular pain and poorly effective for back pain. Thus, a clear understanding of

F. Laroche and S. Perrot (eds.), *Managing Sciatica and Radicular Pain in Primary Care Practice*, DOI: 10.1007/978-1-907673-56-6_7, © Springer Healthcare 2013

the indications for surgery is required. In all cases, psychosocial factors should be considered to avoid poor outcomes.

The situation with respect to cervical radiculopathy is similar to that in the lumbar spine. Although cervical radicular pain often improves without surgery, a significant proportion of patients will require surgical treatment due to persistent severe symptoms [8]; for example, in a population-based study in Rochester, Minnesota, 26% of patients with cervical radiculopathy required surgery during a median follow-up period of 4.9 years [9].

The surgical options available to patients with radiculopathy include discectomy, laminectomy, foraminotomy, vertebral fusion and disc replacement.

Discectomy

Discectomy involves the removal of the herniated part of the central portion, the nucleus pulposus, of an intervertebral disc in order to relieve pressure on a nerve root or the spinal cord. Variations of the discectomy technique include minimally invasive procedures (microdiscectomy) (Figure 7.1) and endoscopic or laser techniques.

Discectomy for lumbar radiculopathy

In patients with radiculopathy associated with a herniated lumbar disc, both open discectomy and microdiscectomy have been shown to be more effective than nonsurgical therapy in terms of short-term (2–3 months) improvements in pain and function [5,10]. For example, in the Spine Outcome Research Trial (SPORT), lumbar discectomy produced greater improvements in pain and physical function than nonsurgical treatment at all time-points up to 1 year, although the differences were not statistically significant and the findings are difficult to interpret due to high non-adherence rates in both groups [11]. The high crossover rate in this trial, with analysis of results on an 'intention to treat' basis probably underestimates the benefit conferred by surgery. Long-term follow-up of the patients in this trial showed that improvements in leg pain and physical function were maintained over 4 years (Figure 7.2) [12]; the proportion of patients who had returned to work by 4 years was similar

Microdiscectomy of a lumbar disc

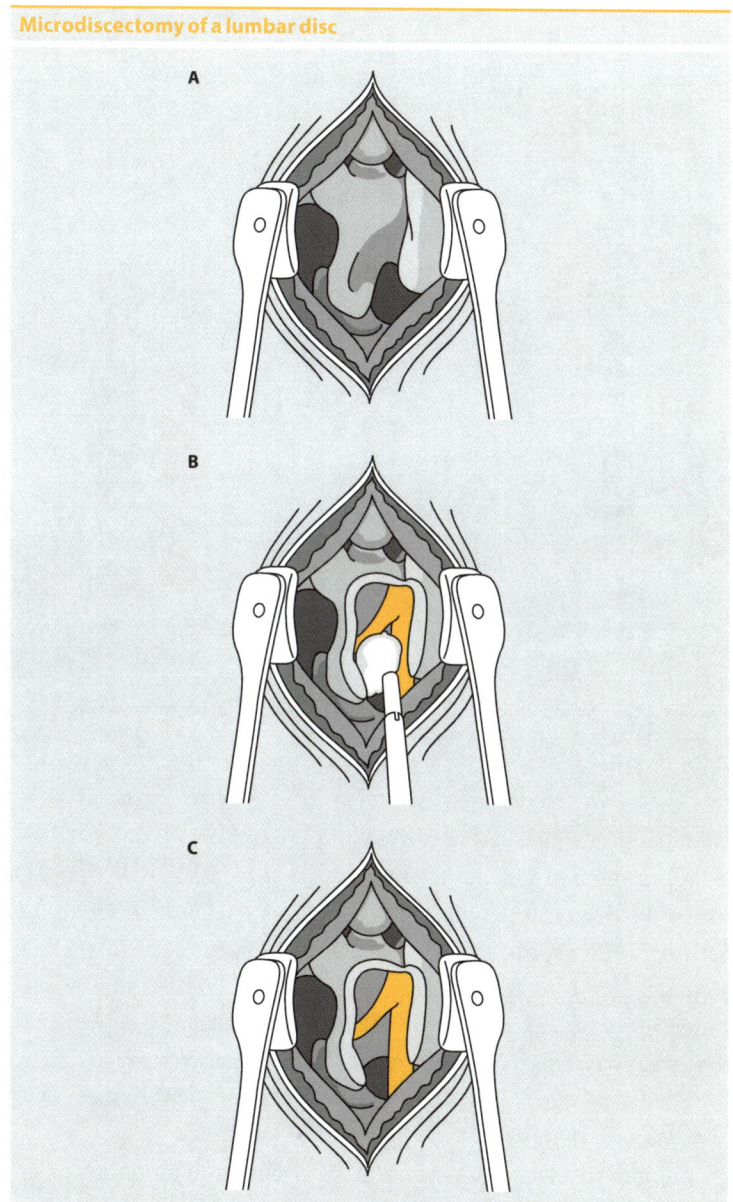

Figure 7.1 Microdiscectomy of a lumbar disc. A, Spine exposed; B, herniated disc material is removed; C, herniated part of the disc has been removed and the nerve root decompressed. Adapted with permission from Buffalo Neurosurgery Group.

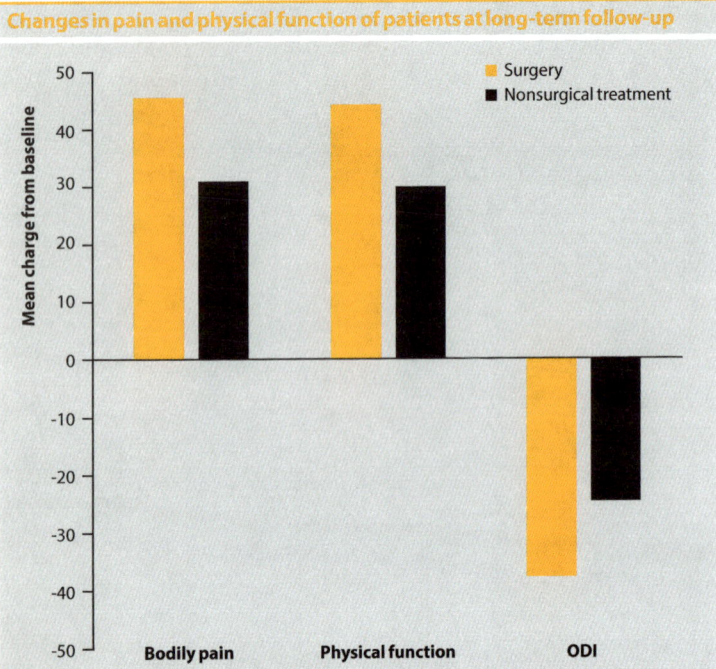

Figure 7.2 Changes in pain and physical function of patients at long-term follow-up.
Changes in Short-form-36 bodily pain and physical function scales and Oswestry Disability Index (ODI) at 4 years in patients with radiculopathy due to a herniated lumbar disc receiving surgical or nonsurgical treatment in the SPORT study. Data from Weinstein et al [12].

in the surgical and nonsurgical treatment groups (84.4% versus 78.4%, respectively) and was not related to improvements in pain, function or satisfaction with treatment [12,13]. Other studies have found that although discectomy results in faster improvements in pain and function in the short-term, there are few significant differences in outcome between surgical and nonsurgical patients after about 1 year [5,13,14]. One study has reported that 1-year outcomes after discectomy in patients who had sciatica symptoms for less than 1 year were better than in those with a longer duration of symptoms [2].

Lumbar discectomy is associated with a low risk of serious complications. In the SPORT study and an accompanying observational cohort study, 95% of open discectomies were free from complications [11,15]. The most common complication associated with discectomy is a dural tear, which has been reported to occur in 1–4% of cases [5,11,14–16]. Re-operation rates for all causes of 3–7% have been reported within 1 year [11,14,15], and 9% within 2 years [11,15].

It remains to be established whether microdiscectomy offers any advantages over non-microscopic procedures in the treatment of lumbar radiculopathy [5,17]. A recent evidence-based review has concluded that the incidence of persistent or recurrent back pain at 2 years is similar with both procedures. A number of studies have failed to find a difference in outcome, length of hospital stay or infection rates whether or not a microscope is used, where reported, the operating time was significantly longer when a microscope was used [18,19,20].

There is currently little published information on the use of endoscopic or laser discectomy techniques [5].

Discectomy for cervical radiculopathy

Cervical radiculopathy is most commonly caused by herniation of a cervical disc [21], which may be treated by either anterior or posterior discectomy [7,21]; anterior discectomy with vertebral fusion (discussed later in this chapter) has traditionally been considered the 'gold standard' of treatment for cervical radiculopathy [21], and posterior discectomy is seldom performed. Current evidence indicates that, although anterior discectomy without fusion can result in spinal instability in some patients [21], functional outcome appears to be comparable with that seen after anterior discectomy with fusion in patients with 1-level radiculopathy; however, fusion may result in more rapid pain reduction and a decreased risk of kyphosis (excessive forward curvature of the spine) [22].

Compared with physical therapy or cervical collar immobilisation, anterior cervical discectomy alone or with fusion can produce greater short-term (3–4 months) improvements in neck or arm pain, weakness and sensory loss in patients with cervical radiculopathy [23]. Furthermore, improvements in motor function in those with weakness at 12 months are greater with anterior discectomy than with physical therapy [23]. However, the success rates in clinical trials vary markedly, from 52% to 99% depending on the patient population studied and the endpoint used, up to 30% of patients may experience recurrent symptoms [23].

One study has reported that patients with electromyographic evidence of nerve root damage before surgery have a better outcome after anterior discectomy with fusion than those without electrophysiological evidence of nerve root involvement [24]; this might suggest that neurophysiological studies could be useful in identifying patients with cervical radiculopathy who could benefit from surgery.

Although anterior cervical discectomy offers advantages over the posterior approach in that the herniated disc can be accessed without compromising nervous tissue [23], it is associated with a number of potential complications. In a retrospective review of 1015 patients undergoing anterior cervical discectomy with fusion [25], the most common complications were dysphagia, which occurred in almost 10% of patients, haematoma and recurrent laryngeal nerve palsy (Table 7.1) [25].

Laminectomy

In the technique of laminectomy, a small piece of bone (the lamina) is removed from one or more vertebrae, in order to relieve pressure on nerve roots or spinal cord (Figure 7.3).

Laminectomy for lumbar radiculopathy

Several studies have shown that lumbar laminectomy improves pain, disability and quality of life in patients with radiculopathy due to lumbar spinal stenosis [26–28], hence laminectomy is now regarded as a mainstay

Complications occurring in patients undergoing anterior cervical discectomy	
Complication	**Number of patients (%)**
Dysphagia	97 (9.5%)
Postoperative haematoma	47 (5.6%)
Recurrent laryngeal nerve palsy	32 (3.1%)
Dural penetration	5 (0.5%)
Oesophageal perforation	3 (0.3%)
Horner's syndrome	1 (0.1%)
Instrument failure	1 (0.1%)

Table 7.1 Complications occurring in patients undergoing anterior cervical discectomy. Complications occurred in 1015 patients undergoing anterior cervical discectomy with fusion for the treatment of cervical radiculopathy, myelopathy or both. Data from Fountas et al [25].

Lumbar laminectomy

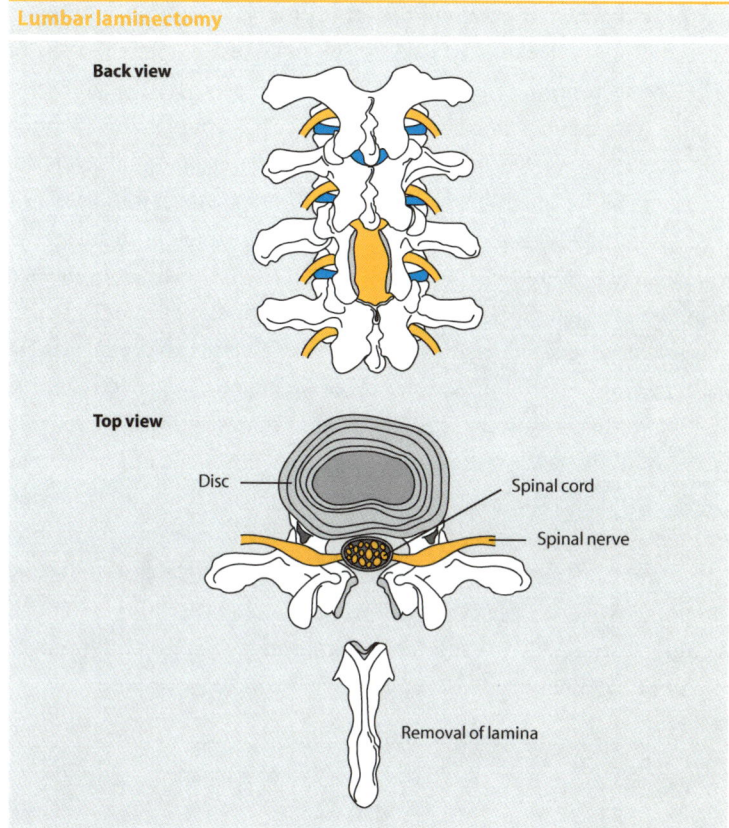

Back view

Top view

Disc

Spinal cord

Spinal nerve

Removal of lamina

Figure 7.3 Lumbar laminectomy.

of treatment for this condition [29]. Long-term success rates of 45–72% have been reported, depending on the endpoint used (leg or back pain, neurological symptoms or ability to work) [28]. Studies comparing laminectomy with conservative management including patient education, exercise and nonsteroidal anti-inflammatory drug (NSAID) treatment, have shown that laminectomy is significantly more effective in relieving pain and improving function [30,31]. In addition, a recent study from the United States has suggested that multilevel laminectomy is cost-effective in the treatment of lumbar stenosis [29]. The available evidence suggests that the incidence of serious complications following lumbar laminectomy is low, but increases with age and comorbidity [28].

Laminectomy for cervical radiculopathy

Laminectomy is commonly used for the treatment of radiculopathy or myelopathy resulting from multilevel cervical spondylysis, a number of studies have demonstrated the efficacy of the procedure in this situation [32–34]. However, it is associated with a number of potential complications, including spinal instability and deformity, particularly kyphosis [32]. Accordingly, many surgeons would choose another technique in the presence of pre-existing kyphosis. Alternative techniques include laminoplasty and skip laminectomy. In laminoplasty the lamina is completely cut on one side and partially cut on the other to produce a flap of bone which can be lifted clear of the spinal cord, thus decompressing it and the nerve roots. The bone flap is then supported by one of a number of different means (Figure 7.4). This technique offers a means of decompressing the cord while preserving spinal stability and reducing the risk of haematoma [32].

Several studies [32,34,35] have shown that both laminectomy and laminoplasty are effective in relieving pain and disability, although laminoplasty requires a shorter hospital stay and appears to produce greater functional improvement at 4 months [32,35].

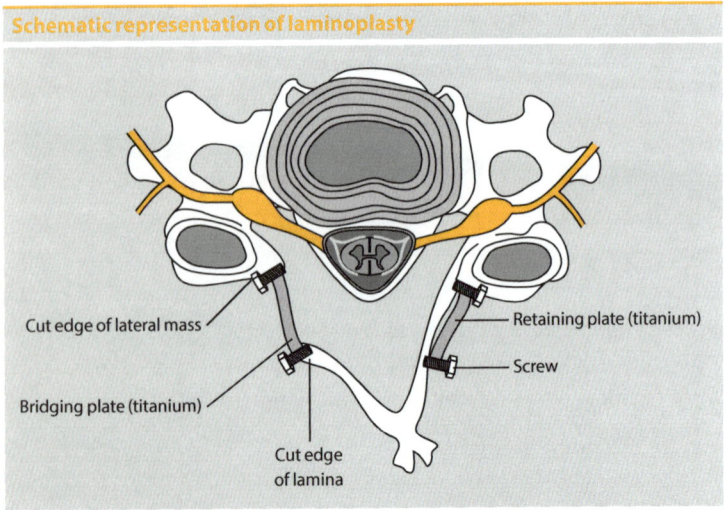

Schematic representation of laminoplasty

Cut edge of lateral mass

Retaining plate (titanium)

Screw

Bridging plate (titanium)

Cut edge of lamina

Figure 7.4 Schematic representation of laminoplasty. Image reproduced with permission from Oxford University Press.

Foraminotomy

Foraminotomy is used to relieve pressure on nerves that are compressed in the intervertebral foramen. This procedure is often performed using minimally invasive techniques [21,36]. Foraminotomy can produce effective relief of cervical radicular pain, there is some evidence that it also improves function, but reported success rates vary widely, from 52–90% [23].

Foraminotomy and laminectomy offer direct visualisation of the nerve root and good exposure of the nerve root exit from the spinal column [8]. However, these procedures are associated with a number of potential complications, including surgical complications, injury to the dura, air embolism and subdural haematoma [8]. Moreover, instability can occur if more than 50% of the facet is excised [8].

Spinal fusion

Fusion may be required in a variety of conditions associated with spinal instability. The criteria for fusion are not universally accepted because the clinical definitions of instability are imprecise [37]. Deformities such as spondylolisthesis and scoliosis are well accepted indications. Fusion is sometimes indicated after a cervical discectomy, especially when there is spondylosis or osteophytes, but is seldom performed after routine lumbar discectomy [37].

For patients with cervical radiculopathy, recommendations for fusion techniques have been published by the American Association of Neurological Surgeons/Congress of Neurological Surgeons (Table 7.2) [22]. Vertebral fusion for cervical radiculopathy can be achieved by various means, including:

- bone auto- or allografts;
- interbody cages; and
- static or dynamic plating.

There is currently insufficient evidence to establish the optimal fusion technique in patients undergoing lumbar surgery [5].

Potential risks associated with fusion procedures include graft site pain and sensory disturbance, graft displacement, implant complications and pseudoarthrosis [8].

American Association of Neurological Surgeons and Congress of Neurological Surgeons recommendations for vertebral fusion in patients with cervical radiculopathy

Recommendation	
Anterior cervical discectomy with fusion is recommended to produce faster reductions in neck and arm pain than discectomy alone in patients with 1-level cervical disc degeneration.	Grade D
• The addition of a cervical plate is recommended if the aim is: – to reduce the risk of pseudoarthrosis and graft problems; and	Grade D
– to maintain lordosis	Grade C
• Cervical arthroplasty is recommended as an alternative to discectomy with fusion to relieve neck or arm pain in selected patients.	Grade B
Anterior discectomy with fusion also decreases the risk of kyphosis, compared with discectomy alone.	Grade C
In patients with 2-level cervical disc degeneration, anterior cervical plating is recommended over discectomy with fusion for the improvement of arm pain.	Grade C
Cervical arthroplasty is recommended as an alternative to discectomy with fusion to relieve neck or arm pain in selected patients.	Grade B

Table 7.2 American Association of Neurological Surgeons and Congress of Neurological Surgeons recommendations for vertebral fusion in patients with cervical radiculopathy. Recommendations are graded A–D in increasing order, according to the strength of the available evidence. Data from Matz et al [22].

Disc replacement

Intervertebral disc replacement with prosthetic discs (spinal arthroplasty) has emerged during the last decade as a means of avoiding the need for vertebral fusion and a variety of such devices are now available [37,38]. Recent systematic reviews have indicated that disc replacement provides comparable results to fusion or fixation techniques, both in lumbar [39] and in cervical [40] surgery. The device must maintain the proper intervertebral spacing, allow for motion and provide stability. However, in both cases only limited long-term data are available. Nevertheless, cervical arthroplasty has been recommended as an alternative to anterior cervical discectomy with fusion to relieve neck and arm pain in selected patients with radiculopathy [22]. A number of different types of disc prosthesis are available, hydrogel disc prosthesis and articulating discs, amongst others. These techniques are best regarded as evolving techniques, or techniques in development. Ultimately they may come to replace intervertebral fusion, but there is a need to compare all available devices, not only on mechanical properties but also on long-term efficacy and stability.

Pain management techniques

Lumbar radicular pain can be considered as a complex pathophysiological condition, which may be treated by pain modulation and pain management techniques. Spinal cord stimulation has been used in lumbar radicular pain, mostly in failed back surgery syndrome, with some efficacy [41].

References

1 Weber H, Holme I, Amlie E. The natural course of acute sciatica with nerve root symptoms in a double-blind placebo-controlled trial evaluating the effect of piroxicam. *Spine.* 1993;18:1433-1438.

2 Ng LC, Sell P. Predictive value of the duration of sciatica for lumbar discectomy. A prospective cohort study. *J Bone Joint Surg Br.* 2004;86:546-549.

3 Koes BW, van Tulder MW, Peul WC. Diagnosis and treatment of sciatica. *BMJ.* 2007;334:1313-1317.

4 Vroomen PC, de Krom MC, Slofstra PD, Knottnerus JA. Conservative treatment of sciatica: a systematic review. *J Spinal Disord.* 2000;13:463-469.

5 Chou R, Baisden J, Carragee EJ, et al. Surgery for low back pain: a review of the evidence for an American Pain Society Clinical Practice Guideline. *Spine.* 2009;34:1094-1109.

6 Chou R, Loeser JD, Owens DK, et al. Interventional therapies, surgery, and interdisciplinary rehabilitation for low back pain: an evidence-based clinical practice guideline from the American Pain Society. *Spine.* 2009;34:1066-1077.

7 Whitney SN, McGuire AL, McCullough LB. A typology of shared decision making, informed consent, and simple consent. *Ann Intern Med.* 2004;140:54-59.

8 Riew KD, Cheng I, Pimenta L, Taylor B. Posterior cervical spine surgery for radiculopathy. *Neurosurgery.* 2007;60:S57-S63.

9 Radhakrishnan K, Litchy WJ, O'Fallon WM, Kurland LT. Epidemiology of cervical radiculopathy. A population-based study from Rochester, Minnesota, 1976 through 1990. *Brain.* 1994;117:325-335.

10 Gibson JN, Waddell G. Surgical interventions for lumbar disc prolapse. *Cochrane Database Syst Rev.* 2007;1:CD001350.

11 Weinstein JN, Tosteson TD, Lurie JD, et al. Surgical vs nonoperative treatment for lumbar disk herniation: the Spine Patient Outcomes Research Trial (SPORT): a randomized trial. *JAMA.* 2006;296:2441-2450.

12 Weinstein JN, Lurie JD, Tosteson TD, et al. Surgical versus nonoperative treatment for lumbar disc herniation: four-year results for the Spine Patient Outcomes Research Trial (SPORT). *Spine.* 2008;33:2789-2800.

13 Valat JP, Genevay S, Marty M, Rozenberg S, Koes B. Sciatica. *Best Pract Res Clin Rheumatol.* 2010;24:241-252.

14 Peul WC, van Houwelingen HC, van den Hout WB, et al. Surgery versus prolonged conservative treatment for sciatica. *N Engl J Med.* 2007;356:2245-2256.

15 Weinstein JN, Lurie JD, Tosteson TD, et al. Surgical vs nonoperative treatment for lumbar disk herniation: the Spine Patient Outcomes Research Trial (SPORT) observational cohort. *JAMA.* 2006;296:2451-2459.

16 Atlas SJ, Deyo RA, Keller RB, et al. The Maine Lumbar Spine Study, Part II. 1-year outcomes of surgical and nonsurgical management of sciatica. *Spine.* 1996;21:1777-1786.

17 Watters WC III, McGirt MJ. An evidence-based review of the literature on the consequences of conservative versus aggressive discectomy for the treatment of primary disc herniation with radiculopathy. *Spine J.* 2009;9:240-257.

18 Gibson JN, Waddell G. Surgical interventions for lumbar disc prolapse: updated Cochrane Review. *Spine*. 2007;32:1735-1747.

19 Türeyen K. One-level one-sided lumbar disc surgery with and without microscopic assistance: 1-year outcome in 114 consecutive patients. *J Neurosurg*. 2003;99;247-250.

20 Katayama et al. Comparison of surgical outcomes between macro discectomy and micro discectomy for lumbar disc herniation: a prospective randomized study with surgery performed by the same spine surgeon. *J Spinal Disord Tech*. 2006;19:344-347.

21 Nasca RJ. Cervical radiculopathy: current diagnostic and treatment options. *J Surg Orthop Adv*. 2009;18:13-18.

22 Matz PG, Ryken TC, Groff MW, et al. Techniques for anterior cervical decompression for radiculopathy. *J Neurosurg Spine*. 2009;11:183-197.

23 Matz PG, Holly LT, Groff MW, et al. Indications for anterior cervical decompression for the treatment of cervical degenerative radiculopathy. *J Neurosurg Spine*. 2009;11:174-182.

24 Alrawi MF, Khalil NM, Mitchell P, Hughes SP. The value of neurophysiogical and imaging studies in predicting outcome in the surgical treatment of cervical radiculopathy. *Eur Spine J*. 2007;16:495-500.

25 Fountas KN, Kapsalaki EZ, Nikolakakos LG, et al. Anterior cervical discectomy and fusion associated complications. *Spine*. 2007;32:2310-2317.

26 Gibson JN, Waddell G. Surgery for degenerative lumbar spondylosis: updated Cochrane Review. *Spine*. 2005;30:2312-2320.

27 Weinstein JN, Lurie JD, Olson PR, Bronner KK, Fisher ES. United States' trends and regional variations in lumbar spine surgery: 1992-2003. *Spine*. 2006;31:2707-2714.

28 Genevay S, Atlas SJ. Lumbar spinal stenosis. *Best Pract Res Clin Rheumatol*. 2010;24:253-265.

29 Parker SL, Fulchiero EC, Davis BJ, et al. Cost-effectiveness of multilevel hemilaminectomy for lumbar stenosis-associated radiculopathy. *Spine J*. 2011;11:705-711.

30 Malmivaara A, Slätis P, Heliövaara M, et al. Surgical or nonoperative treatment for lumbar spinal stenosis? A randomized controlled trial. *Spine*. 2007;32:1-8.

31 Weinstein JN, Tosteson TD, Lurie JD, et al. Surgical versus nonsurgical therapy for lumbar spinal stenosis. *N Engl J Med*. 2008;358:794-810.

32 Kaminsky SB, Clark CR, Traynelis VC. Operative treatment of cervical spondylotic myelopathy and radiculopathy. A comparison of laminectomy and laminoplasty at five year average follow-up. *Iowa Orthop J*. 2004;24:95-105.

33 Clark CR. Indications and surgical management of cervical myelopathy. *Sem Spine Surg*. 1989;1:254-261.

34 Nakano N, Nakano T, Nakano K. Comparison of the results of laminectomy and open-door laminoplasty for cervical spondylotic myeloradiculopathy and ossification of the posterior longitudinal ligament. *Spine*. 1988;13:792-794.

35 Hardman J, Graf O, Kouloumberis PE, et al. Clinical and functional outcomes of laminoplasty and laminectomy. *Neurol Res*. 2010;32:416-420.

36 Jho HD. Microsurgical anterior cervical foraminotomy for radiculopathy: a new approach to cervical disc herniation. *J Neurosurg*. 1996;84:155-160.

37 Mayer HM. Total lumbar disc replacement. *J Bone Joint Surg Br*. 2005;87:1029-1037.

38 Phillips FM, Garfin SR. Cervical disc replacement. *Spine*. 2005;30:S27-S33.

39 van den Eerenbeemt KD, Ostelo RW, van Royen BJ, Peul WC, van Tulder MW. Total disc replacement surgery for symptomatic degenerative lumbar disc disease: a systematic review of the literature. *Eur Spine J*. 2010;19:1262-1280.

40 Zechmeister I, Winkler R, Mad P. Artificial total disc replacement versus fusion for the cervical spine: a systematic review. *Eur Spine J*. 2011;20:177-184.

41 Frey ME, Manchikanti L, Benyamin RM, Schultz DM, Smith HS, Cohen SP. Spinal cord stimulation for patients with failed back surgery syndrome: a systematic review. *Pain Physician*. 2009;12:379-397.

Development of this book was supported by funding from Pfizer

Chapter 8

Pharmacological treatment options available for radicular pain

Paolo Marchettini

As described in Chapter 5, various forms of pharmacological therapy may be indicated in patients with sciatica [1–4] and other forms of radiculopathy [5,6]. The primary aim of pharmacological therapy in patients with radicular pain is analgesia; as with other conservative measures, drug therapy does not generally alter the course of the underlying condition [2]. Pharmacological treatment in patients with radicular pain should form part of a comprehensive treatment programme, tailored to the needs of the individual patient, which includes conservative management and physical therapy as appropriate, with referral for possible surgery if symptoms remain uncontrolled.

Paracetamol

Patients with sciatica are likely to first turn to readily available agents for pain relief, such as paracetamol either with or without codeine. Paracetamol is currently recommended as first-line analgesic therapy in the Dutch guidelines for the treatment of sciatica resulting from radiculopathy [1,2] and the American College of Physicians/American Pain Society (ACP/APS) guidelines for the management of low back pain (LBP) [3,4]. Studies in patients with LBP, including pain due to radiculopathy, have yielded moderate evidence that paracetamol is more effective than placebo in providing short-term (≤4 weeks) pain relief [4]. However, in

F. Laroche and S. Perrot (eds.), *Managing Sciatica and Radicular Pain in Primary Care Practice*, DOI: 10.1007/978-1-907673-56-6_8, © Springer Healthcare 2013

patients with chronic back pain, paracetamol has been reported to be less effective as an analgesic than the nonsteroidal anti-inflammatory drug (NSAID) diflunisal [7]. This is consistent with the findings of systematic reviews in patients with osteoarthritis, which have consistently shown paracetamol to be less effective than NSAIDs [4,8–11].

Paracetamol is generally well tolerated. The most common adverse events include gastrointestinal disturbances and headache, the incidences of which appear to be similar with sustained-release and immediate-release formulations [12]. However, there is also a well-documented risk of liver damage when paracetamol is taken in overdose. Indeed, paracetamol overdose is the most common cause of acute liver failure in some Western countries [13]. Furthermore, it should be noted that there are few data on the risk of serious adverse events, including hepatic toxicity and gastrointestinal bleeding, in patients receiving paracetamol for the treatment of sciatica [4].

Paracetamol plus codeine may also be used to help manage sciatica pain. It is available over the counter in certain countries, though in the United States it is only available with a prescription. However, it should only be used in the short term and patients may experience the side effects associated with opioids, such as drowsiness and nausea [14].

Nonsteroidal anti-inflammatory drugs

Nonsteroidal anti-inflammatory drugs are recommended as second-line analgesics in the Dutch guidelines [1,2] and as first-line treatment in the ACP/APS guidelines [3,4]. Previous systematic reviews have found no evidence to support the use of NSAIDs in the treatment of sciatica [2,15–17], but in a more recent Cochrane review, NSAIDs were slightly but significantly more effective than placebo in producing short-term (≤3 weeks) reductions in pain intensity (mean treatment difference –8.39, 95% confidence interval [CI] –12.68, –4.10) and the proportion of patients with acute LBP experiencing global improvement (risk ratio [RR] 1.19, 95% CI 1.07, 1.33). They were also significantly more effective than placebo in reducing chronic low back pain (cLBP; mean treatment difference –12.40, 95% CI –15.53, –9.26) [18]. There were no significant differences in efficacy, in terms of pain reductions or global improvements, between NSAIDs and paracetamol, or between NSAIDs and other drugs, including narcotic analgesics and muscle relaxants [18]. Treatment with NSAIDs was associated with a significantly higher incidence of adverse events, compared with placebo (acute back pain: RR 1.35, 95% CI 1.09, 1.68; chronic back pain: RR 1.24, 95% CI 1.07, 1.43) or paracetamol (RR 1.76, 95% CI 1.12, 2.76). Cyclooxygenase-2 (COX-2)-specific inhibitors were comparable in analgesic efficacy to nonselective NSAIDs in patients with acute LBP (mean treatment difference –1.17, 95% CI –4.67, 2.33), and were associated with a lower risk of adverse events (RR 0.83, 95% CI 0.70, 0.99) [18]. There was no evidence that any nonselective NSAID was superior in efficacy to the others.

Nonsteroidal anti-inflammatory drugs are associated with a number of well-documented adverse events (Table 8.1) [19], including gastrointestinal disturbances such as dyspepsia or nausea and alterations in renal function. Such adverse events are usually mild or moderate in severity [18], although serious gastrointestinal complications such as bleeding or ulceration can occur [19]. Selective COX-2 inhibitors are associated with a lower risk of gastrointestinal adverse events than nonselective agents [20]; however, some of these agents are associated with an increased risk of cardiovascular adverse events [20,21], although it is unclear whether this is a significant concern during the short treatment periods recommended for sciatica [18].

Adverse events associated with NSAIDs
Gastrointestinal disturbances such as abdominal pain or diarrhoea
Oedema
Dry mouth
Rash
Dizziness
Headache
Tiredness
Alterations in renal function
Platelet inhibition resulting in bleeding

Table 8.1 Adverse events associated with NSAIDs. Data adapted from Roelofs et al [18] and Ong et al [19].

Nonsteroidal anti-inflammatory drugs for neuropathic pain

While NSAIDs are effective against nociceptive pain, they have very limited success at alleviating the neuropathic component of radicular pain, often expressed as pain in the lower limb [22,23]. They work best when there is an inflammatory component, which is not present in neuropathic pain [22,24,25]. Nevertheless, they are widely prescribed for patients with neuropathic pain disorders, including LBP. Possible reasons for the widespread use of NSAIDs despite their lack of efficacy in these cases include their low cost and easy availability and physicians' comfort level with them [26].

Opioids

Several currently available potential pharmacological options for the treatment of the neuropathic component of radicular pain are listed in Table 8.2 [27]. However, it is important to note that in the European Union only tramadol, the opioid agonists and pregabalin are approved for use in radicular pain.

Opioid agonists, such as morphine and oxycodone, have been prescribed by primary care physicians for the treatment of LBP for several years. A survey conducted in the United States from 1995 to 1998 in over 25,000 patients with spinal and radicular pain found that 3.4% had opioids included in their treatment plans. Those who had pain symptoms for longer than 3 months and/or who had pain due to injury or a herniated disc were more likely to prescribed opioids [28].

Clinical trials have investigated the efficacy of long-acting versus short-acting opioids for the treatment of persistent, moderate-to-severe back pain. In one study, 47 patients were randomised to receive 5 mg of immediate-release oxycodone four times daily or 10 mg of controlled-release oxycodone every 12 hours, with titration up to 80 mg/day, for up to 10 days and then crossed over to the other treatment for 4 to 7 days. Ninety-one percent of patients achieved stable analgesia with no significant differences in overall pain intensity between treatments. Nearly all reported adverse events were mild to moderate; the most common were constipation, somnolence, dizziness, nausea and pruritus [29].

Another randomised study compared extended-release oxymorphone (titrated at 10–110 mg every 12 hours), controlled-release oxymorphone (titrated at 20–220 mg every 12 hours) and placebo in 330 patients. Once the opioid doses were stable, patients received that treatment or placebo for 18 days. Treatment with both formulations of oxymorphone led to greater mean changes in pain intensity from baseline than placebo ($P=0.0001$). Significantly more patients taking oxymorphone rated their drug as "good", "very good" or "excellent". Most adverse events were mild to moderate and there was no difference in the rate of adverse events between oxymorphone formulations [30].

An analysis of data from 26,000 patients found that longer opioid use was associated with greater rates of mental health conditions (eg, depression, anxiety). Sixty-one percent of patients had been prescribed an opioid within a year of their first visit for LBP, with 19% of that group having at least one course of opioid therapy lasting 120 days or longer. Approximately 60% of the patients long-term opioid use were given short-acting agents; the other 40% were given a mix of long- and short-acting opioids [31].

Tramadol is an agonist of the opioid μ-receptor with similar efficacy and side effects as opioids. However, because tramadol inhibits serotonin and norepinephrine reuptake, it may precipitate the serotonin syndrome if given in combination with selective serotonin reuptake inhibitors (SSRI) or selective norepinephrine reuptake inhibitors (SNRI). Both tramadol and other opioids should be considered as second-line therapy for LBP [27].

Tapentadol is a centrally acting analgesic with a dual mode of action as an agonist of the μ-opioid receptor and as a norepinephrine reuptake inhibitor [32]. While its analgesic actions have been compared to tramadol and oxycodone [33], its general potency is somewhere between tramadol and morphine in effectiveness. Like tramadol, in combination with SSRIs or SNRIs and/or monoamine oxidase inhibitors it may cause serotonin syndrome [34].

For chronic low back pain, strong opioids should not be prescribed except in very specific cases (including a strict contract with the patient) and preferentially initiated by pain specialists [35].

Principal pharmacological options for the treatment of radicular pain

Medication class	Starting dosage	Titration	Maximum dosage
Calcium channel α2-δ ligands • Gabapentin	100–300 mg at bedtime or 100–300 mg three times daily	Increase by 100–300 mg three times daily every 1–7 days, as tolerated, until pain relief	3600 mg daily (1200 mg three times daily); reduce if impaired renal function
• Pregabalin	50 mg three times daily or 75 mg twice daily	Increase to 300 mg daily after 3–7 days, then by 150 mg/day every 3–7 days, as tolerated, until pain relief	600 mg daily (200 mg 3 times daily or 300 mg twice daily); reduce if impaired renal function
Secondary amine TCAs • Nortriptyline[†] • Desipramine[†]	25 mg at bedtime	Increase by 25 mg daily every 3–7 days, as tolerated, until pain relief	150 mg daily; if blood level of active drug and its metabolite is <100 ng/mL (mg/mL), continue titration with caution
Opioid agonists* • Morphine, oxycodone, methadone, levorphanol[†]	10–15 mg morphine every 4 hours or as needed (equianalgesic dosages should be used for other opioid analgesics)	After 1–2 weeks, convert total daily dosage to long-acting opioid analgesic and continue short-acting medication as needed	No maximum dosage with careful titration; consider evaluation by pain specialist at relatively high dosages (eg, 120–180 mg morphine daily; equianalgesic dosages should be used for other opioid analgesics)
• Tramadol[‡]	50 mg once or twice daily	Increase by 50–100 mg daily in divided doses every 3–7 days, as tolerated, until pain relief	400 mg daily (100 mg four times daily); in patients age >75 years, 300 mg daily
• Tapentadol	50 mg twice daily	Increase to 50 mg twice daily every 7 days	250 mg twice daily

Table 8.2 Principal pharmacological options for the treatment of radicular pain. SNRI, selective norepinephrine reuptake inhibitor; SSRI, selective serotonin reuptake inhibitor; TCA, tricyclic antidepressant (use tertiary amine TCA if a secondary amine TCA is not available). *First-line only in certain circumstances; [†]consider lower starting dosages and slower titration in geriatric patients; [‡]consider lower starting dosages and slower titration in geriatric patients, dosages given are for short-acting formulation. Adapted from O'Connor & Dworkin [27].

Duration of adequate trial	Major side effects	Precautions	Other benefits
3–8 weeks for titration + 2 weeks at maximum dose	Sedation, dizziness, peripheral oedema	Renal insufficiency	Improvement of sleep disturbance, no clinically significant drug interactions
4 weeks	Sedation, dizziness, peripheral oedema	Renal insufficiency	Improvement of sleep disturbance, improvement of anxiety, no clinically significant drug interaction
6–8 weeks with ≥2 weeks at maximum tolerated dosage	Sedation, dry mouth, blurred vision, weight gain, urinary retention	Cardiac disease, glaucoma, suicide risk, seizure disorder, concomitant use of tramadol	Improvement of depression, improvement of insomnia, low cost
4–6 weeks	Nausea/vomiting, constipation, drowsiness, dizziness, tolerance over time	History of substance abuse, suicide risk, driving impairment during treatment initiation. Strong opioids should be prescribed only when all other pain medication fail to provide relief, they should not be first-line treatment	Rapid onset of analgesic benefit
4 weeks	Nausea/vomiting, constipation, drowsiness, dizziness, seizures	History of substance abuse, suicide risk, driving impairment during treatment initiation, seizure disorder, concomitant use of SSRI, SNRI or TCA	Rapid onset of analgesic benefit
5 weeks	Nausea, dizziness, headache, dry mouth, fatigue, constipation, diarrhea, nasopharyngitis, somnolence	Epilepsy, lung disease, kidney disease, history of drug or alcohol abuse, also negative drug interactions with sleep and antipsychotic drugs	Reduced GI adverse events compared to oxycodone

Tricyclic antidepressants

The ACP/APS guidelines recommend tricyclic antidepressants (TCAs) as a short-term option in patients with LBP who have no contraindications to their use [3,4]. Other classes of antidepressants do not have proven efficacy for LBP relief [36]. However, the effects of TCAs are only small to moderate [4].

In one study of the TCA nortriptyline vs. placebo for relief of cLBP (n=78), a 22% decrease in pain intensity was noted with nortriptyline compared with 9% for placebo (*P*=0.05). Treatment with nortriptyline led to a nonsignificant reduction in disability [37]. Another study compared the efficacy of morphine alone, nortriptyline alone, morphine + nortriptyline in combination and placebo in 28 patients with lumbar radicular pain. There were no significant differences in leg pain or LBP scores among any of the therapies. During the last 2 weeks of maintenance therapy, the patients taking nortriptyline alone experienced a 14% reduction in average leg pain versus placebo, compared with a 7% reduction seen in the morphine alone and the combination groups [38].

The decision to prescribe TCAs for radicular pain should take into account the adverse events associated with these medications. Common adverse events seen with TCAs include dry mouth, constipation, fatigue, dizziness and insomnia [38,39].

Calcium channel α2-δ ligands

Gabapentin

Gabapentin is a structural analogue of the inhibitory neurotransmitter γ-aminobutyric acid (GABA) which binds to the α_2- subunit of presynaptic, voltage-dependent, calcium channels [40]. Gabapentin has both anticonvulsant and analgesic properties [40] and it has been shown to be effective in the treatment of neuropathic pain [41,42]. However, comparatively few studies have investigated the efficacy of gabapentin in patients with radiculopathy. In a placebo-controlled study in patients with chronic radiculopathy, gabapentin was found to produce significant improvements in pain, motor function and neurological tests at doses of 900 to 3600 mg/day [43]. A further, open-label, study in patients with chronic lumbosacral radiculopathy found significant improvements in quality of life, disability and depression, compared with baseline levels, after 8 weeks of gabapentin treatment [44]. Short-term (3 months) treatment with gabapentin has also been reported to improve pain and function in patients with radiculopathy due to lumbar spinal stenosis or lumbar disc herniation [45].

Adverse events are common during gabapentin treatment. A recent systematic review of 29 studies of gabapentin ($\geq$1200 mg/day) in patients with neuropathic pain found that adverse events occurred in 66% of patients and 12% of patients discontinued treatment because of adverse events. The most common adverse events were dizziness and somnolence (Figure 8.1) [42].

Pregabalin

Pregabalin is also an analogue of GABA and is a structural analogue of gabapentin [46,47]. It acts in the same way as gabapentin [48] and has been shown to inhibit the release of various neurotransmitters involved in pain pathways, including glutamic acid, noradrenaline, serotonin, dopamine and substance P [46]. Pregabalin has the benefit of linear

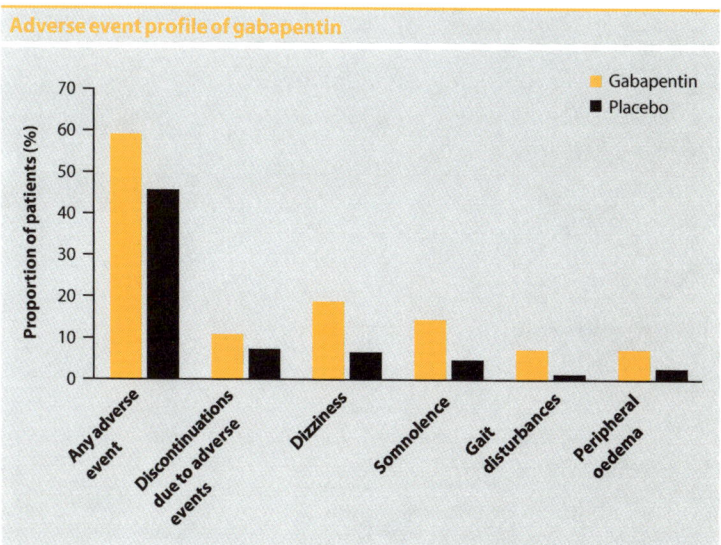

Figure 8.1 Adverse event profile of gabapentin. Use of gabapentin in randomised double-blind trials in patients with neuropathic pain or fibromyalgia. Data from Moore et al [42].

pharmacokinetics [49], allowing for easier dose control [48]. The dosing for pregabalin is twice daily and it has a 6-fold higher affinity for the α2-δ subunit of the voltage-gated calcium channel than gabapentin [48]. In clinical trials, pregabalin has been shown to be effective in the treatment of neuropathic pain, including diabetic neuropathy, postherpetic neuralgia and central pain, and is recommended as first-line treatment for these conditions [41].

Several clinical trials have investigated the efficacy of pregabalin in the treatment of lumbar or cervical radicular pain. In one study, conducted in a primary care setting, 1304 patients with cervical or lumbosacral radiculopathy were treated with pregabalin, alone or in combination with other analgesics, or alternative analgesics for 12 weeks; all patients had

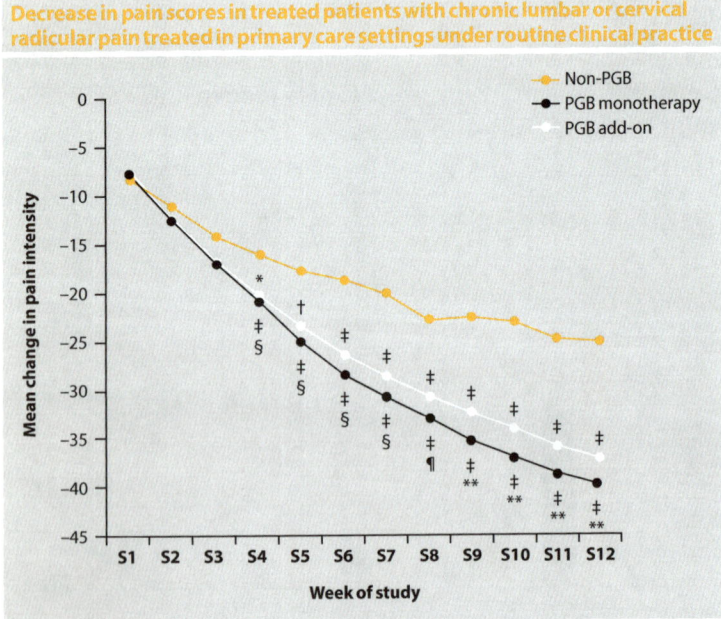

Decrease in pain scores in treated patients with chronic lumbar or cervical radicular pain treated in primary care settings under routine clinical practice

Figure 8.2 Decrease in pain scores in treated patients with chronic lumbar or cervical radicular pain treated in primary care settings under routine clinical practice. Decrease in pain scores, measured on a 100 mm visual analogue scale, in patients with chronic lumbar or cervical radicular pain treated with pregabalin (PBG) alone or in combination with other analgesics, and in patients who did not receive pregabalin (non-PGB). The observed greater pain reduction of the monotherapy group is probably a reflection of the pregabalin add-on group presenting with more severe symptoms. *,†,‡$P<0.05$, <0.01, <0.001 versus non-PGB group; §,¶,**$P<0.05$, <0.01, <0.001 versus PGB add-on. Data from Saldaña et al [50].

experienced chronic neuropathic pain for at least 6 months, which was refractory to previous analgesic therapy [50]. The study was conducted under real-world conditions, meaning that the treatment administered was decided by the physician on the basis of the patient's condition rather than by randomisation [50]. The mean daily pregabalin doses were 187 mg in the monotherapy group and 191 mg in the combination therapy group. Compared with patients who did not receive pregabalin, both the monotherapy and combination therapy groups showed significantly greater reductions from baseline in pain and improvements in health-related quality of life (Figures 8.2 and 8.3) [50]. The observed greater pain reduction of the monotherapy group is probably a reflection of the pregabalin add-on group presenting with more severe symptoms. The mean pain reductions were 56% in patients receiving pregabalin

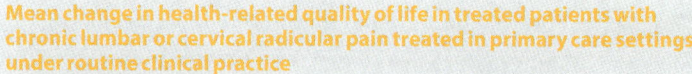

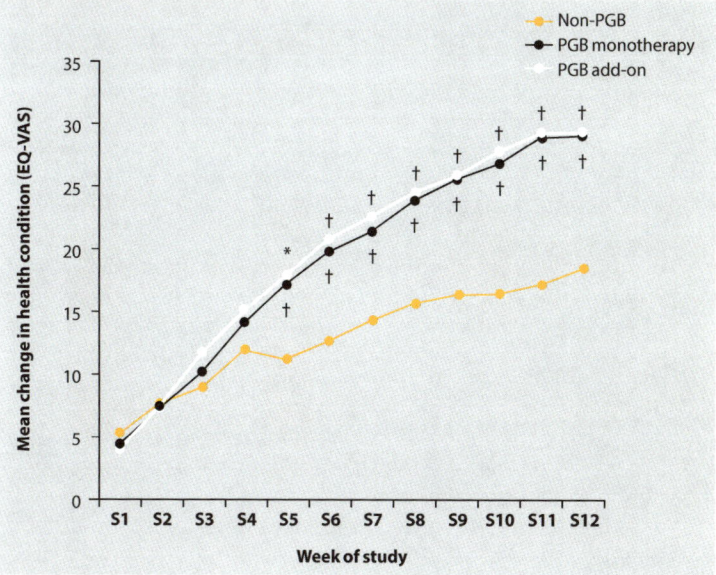

Figure 8.3 Mean change in health-related quality of life in treated patients with chronic lumbar or cervical radicular pain treated in primary care settings under routine clinical practice. The mean change was measured using the EQ-5D visual analogue scale, in patients treated with pregabalin (PGB) alone or in combination with other analgesics, and in patients who did not receive PGB (non-PGB). *,† P<0.01, <0.001 versus non-PGB group. Data from Saldaña et al [50].

monotherapy and 51% in those receiving combination therapy, compared with 36% in patients who did not receive pregabalin ($P<0.0001$). The differences in pain reduction were significant by the fourth week and remained significant for the duration of the study. Pregabalin-treated patients also showed significant improvements in a number of other outcomes, including pain-related depression, anxiety and sleep disturbances, compared with the non-pregabalin group [50].

This study also investigated the impact of pregabalin therapy on health care resource use and treatment costs (Figure 8.4) [51]. Compared with pre-treatment levels, mean drug costs increased significantly ($P<0.001$) more with both pregabalin monotherapy (mean increase €148.60) or combination therapy (€145.30) than with non-pregabalin analgesics (€15.40). However, this was offset by significant reductions in other medical costs and non-medical costs, such that the decrease in total treatment costs was significantly greater with either pregabalin regimen than with non-pregabalin therapy [51]. In a further study in patients

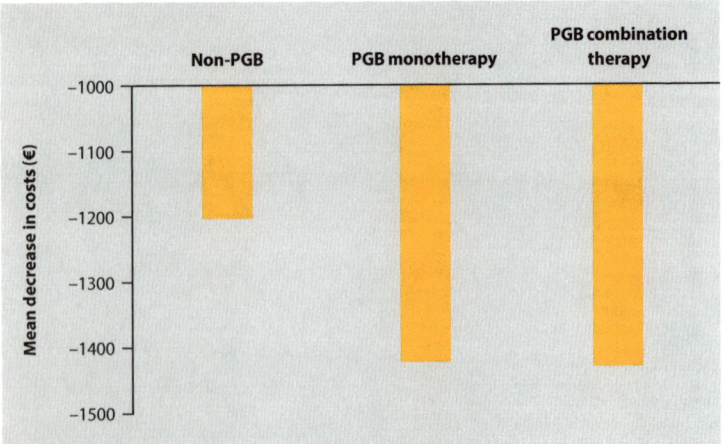

Figure 8.4 Mean reductions in total treatment costs in patients with lumbar or cervical radiculopathy treated in primary care settings under routine clinical practice. The mean reductions in total treatment costs include non-medical costs from pretreatment levels in patients treated with pregabalin (PGB), alone or as monotherapy, or non-PGB analgesics. $P<0.001$ for between-group comparisons. Data from Saldaña et al [51].

with chronic lumbosacral radiculopathy, 58% of patients showed pain reductions of at least 30% during single-blind pregabalin treatment, but there was no significant difference in the time to loss of response between pregabalin-treated and placebo-treated patients [52].

Similar results have been seen in other studies. Investigators conducted a post-hoc analysis of a 6-week observational study of pregabalin for neuropathic pain, reviewing data from the diabetic neuropathic pain, cancer-related neuropathic pain and neuropathic back pain (n=8778). The mean pain scores for each group significantly decreased over the entire 6 weeks. Pain scores improved in the back pain group by 58% [53]. A 12-week, prospective, double-blind trial assessed the efficacy and safety of pregabalin alone, the COX-2 specific inhibitor celecoxib alone and their combination in the treatment of cLBP (n=36). When patients were pooled by Leeds Assessment of Neuropathic Symptoms and Signs (LANSS) score, both pregabalin and celecoxib therapy alone led to significant reductions in pain. However, the combination of pregabalin + celecoxib was more effective in reducing pain in the overall patient population [54].

Pregabalin treatment is generally well tolerated. The most common adverse events are dose-dependent dizziness and somnolence, which are usually mild-to-moderate and transient [46,55], weight gain can also be a side effect. In an analysis of the pooled data from 11 trials in patients with neuropathic pain (diabetic neuropathy or postherpetic neuropathy), the adverse event profile of pregabalin was comparable in elderly (age ≥65 years) and younger patients [55].

Epidural steroids

Epidural corticosteroid injections can be given via the interlaminar (or translaminar), caudal or transforaminal routes (Figure 8.5), depending on the location and source of pain:

- In the interlaminar approach, the injection is given between the lamina of two adjacent vertebrae.
- In the caudal approach, injections are given via the sacrococcygeal membrane.
- In the transforaminal periradicular approach, the injection is given laterally, via the neural foramen.

Epidural corticosteroid injections

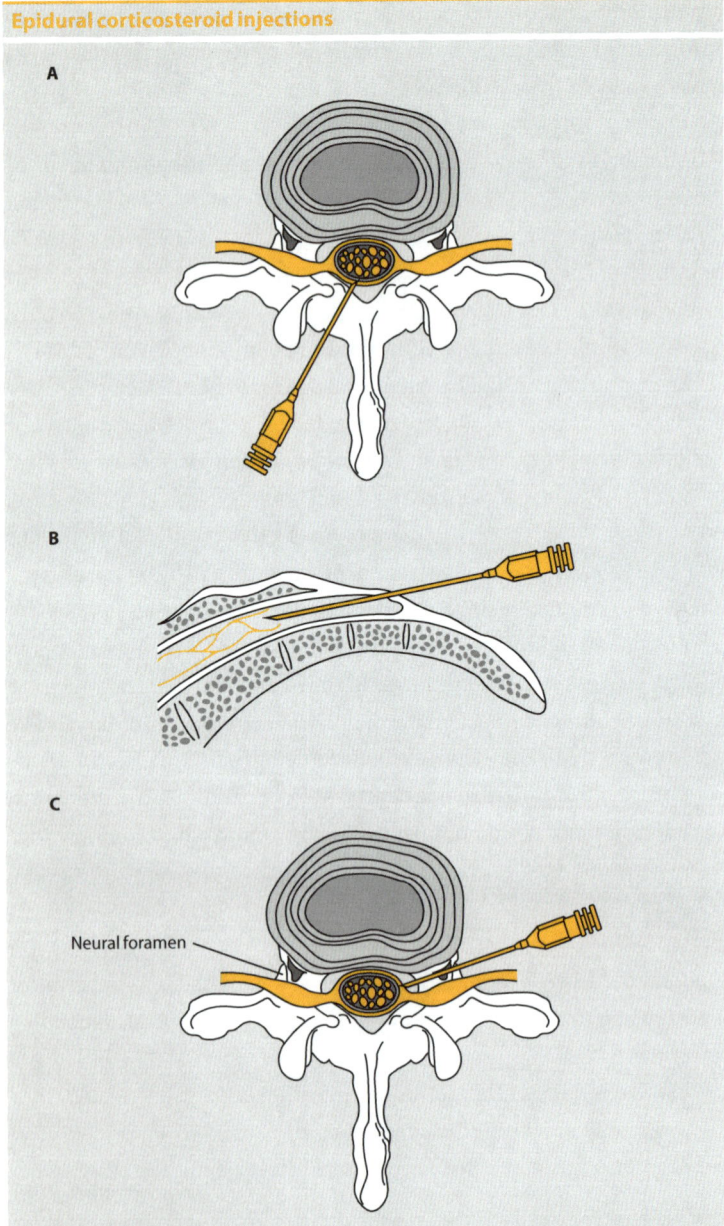

Figure 8.5 Epidural corticosteroid injections. A, Inter(trans)laminar injection; B, caudal injection; C, transforaminal injection.

Epidural injections are given with local anaesthesia, often under radiological guidance. Epidural steroid injections are often used by orthopaedists, anaesthetists and other specialists in the treatment of LBP, and are recommended for short-term (<6 months) pain relief in patients with radiculopathy due to lumbar spinal stenosis [56]. However, a systematic review of studies with epidural injections in patients with lumbosacral radiculopathy found that there was conflicting evidence for short-term (<3 months) efficacy, and that the effects of long-term treatment on disability and return to work were unknown [57]. For these reasons, epidural steroid injections are not recommended for the treatment of sciatica due to radicular pain [57].

About one-third of all epidural steroid injections are given for the treatment of lumbar spinal stenosis [58]. However, studies in this setting have yielded conflicting results, depending on the patient population and injection technique used. In general, interlaminar injections have shown only limited benefit during either short-term or long-term treatment [58,59]. By contrast, in a systematic review of studies in patients with cLBP, including pain due to radiculopathy resulting from lumbar disc herniation or lumbar spinal stenosis, caudal epidural injections were found to reduce pain by at least 50% during both short-term (<6 months) and long-term (1 year) treatment [58,60]. Several studies have suggested that the use of fluoroscopy to guide caudal or transforaminal steroid injections improves the accuracy of delivery, resulting in good medium-term (3 to 36 months) pain relief [56].

Epidural steroid injections have also been used in patients with cervical radiculopathy in whom non-interventional treatments have been unsuccessful [61]. Systematic reviews have shown that such treatment produces short-term pain relief [62], there is some evidence that steroid injection is more effective in patients with herniated discs than in those with spinal stenosis [63]. Evidence for long-term benefits of epidural steroid injections in patients with cervical radiculopathy is limited [62]. However, a recent study has reported that interlaminar or transforaminal steroid injection averted the need for surgery in 79 of 98 patients (80.6%) who were considered surgical candidates, there was no difference in long-term outcome between patients who underwent surgery and those who did not [64].

Potential complications of epidural steroid injections
Increased pain
Injection-site pain
Numbness
Damage to surrounding structures • haematoma • nerve damage
Postdural puncture headache
Arachnoiditis secondary to intrathecal injection
Epidural abscess
Meningitis
Hypercorticism
Allergy

Table 8.3 Potential complications of epidural steroid injections. Data from [65–69].

Epidural steroid injections are associated with a number of potential complications (Table 8.3), including pain, damage to surrounding tissues, postdural puncture headache (PDPH), and rare complications such as epidural abscess or meningitis; in addition, arachnoiditis can occur due to inadvertent intrathecal injection [65–68]. In general, the incidence of such complications appears to be low in patients receiving epidural steroids for the treatment of LBP: in a study involving 228 patients with sciatica, only one case of PDPH was observed following epidural steroid injection [67]. Similarly, minor adverse events have been reported to occur in 5 to 20% of patients after cervical epidural injections, whereas the incidence of major complications is less than 1% [62]. In a retrospective review of 1857 patients who received either lumbar or cervical epidural steroid injections, the overall incidence of minor complications such as injection site pain was 2.4%, and no major complications were recorded. Complications were more common in patients receiving interlaminar injections than in those receiving transforaminal injections (6.0% versus 2.1%, respectively) [69].

Transforaminal periradicular injections
Several studies have reported that transforaminal periradicular steroid injection relieves pain in patients with sciatica [17,70–72], and there is

evidence that this route of administration results in more effective pain relief than the interlaminar approach [73,74]. As noted above, transforaminal injection has been reported to produce good medium-term pain relief in patients with radiculopathy due to lumbar spinal stenosis [56]. There is also evidence from systematic reviews that transforaminal injection can produce long-term pain relief in patients with either lumbar or cervical radiculopathy [75], but there is a risk of severe complications, including irreversible spinal cord injury [76].

As with other routes of epidural injection, the incidence of serious complications is generally considered to be low with transforaminal lumbar injection [62,67,69]. However, one study has reported 78 major complications following cervical transforaminal injections, including infarctions (some fatal) involving the cerebellum, brainstem or posterior cerebral artery territory [76]. These complications were attributed to embolism, vertebral artery perforation or needle-induced vasospasm. It should be noted however, that this was a retrospective questionnaire study and the response rate was low (21.4%) [76].

Systemic steroids

Intravenous (IV) and intramuscular (IM) steroid injections can quickly deliver large doses of medication to the affected areas [77]. However, their efficacy for LBP has not been proven in clinical trials.

One randomised study looked at the effect of a single IV glucocorticoid bolus on acute discogenic sciatica symptoms. Sixty patients were given either placebo or 500 mg of methylprednisolone and followed for 30 days. Evolution of leg pain significantly decreased in the steroid group during the first 3 days following treatment administration (P=0.04 vs placebo); results were similar between groups from Days 3–30. No differences were seen in improvement of pain during the first 10 days and other secondary outcomes [77].

Another placebo-controlled, randomised study assessed a single IM injection of methylprednisolone as adjunctive treatment for non-radicular LBP (n=87). Patients treated in the emergency room for LBP were given the injection before discharge and followed up 1 month later. At 1 month, there was a non-significant difference in change in numerical rating scores

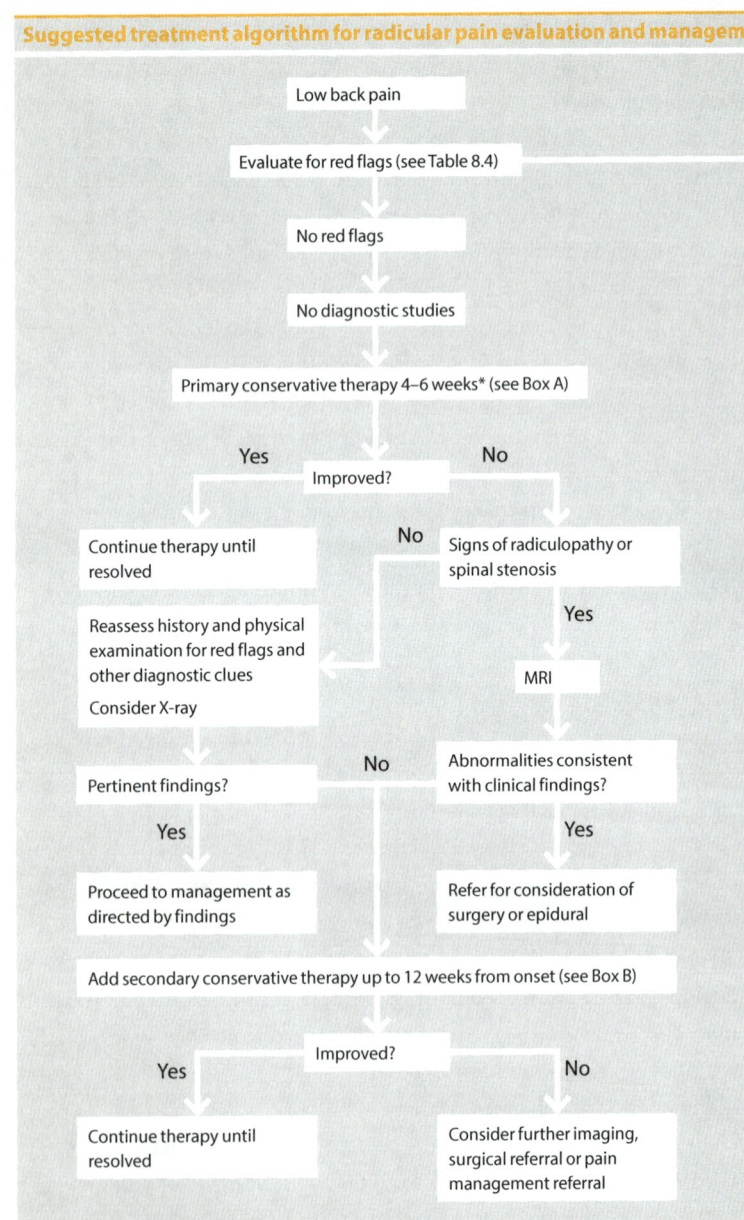

Figure 8.6 Suggested treatment algorithm for radicular pain evaluation and management.
CBC, complete blood count; CT, computed tomography; ESR, erythrocyte sedimentation rate;
CRP, C-reactive protein; NSAIDs, nonsteroidal anti-inflammatory drugs; MRI, magnetic resonance
imaging; TCA, tricyclic antidepressants. Data from Duffy [79]. © 2010, with permission from Elsevier.

Red flags suggest:

Cauda equina syndrome	Fracture	Infection	Neoplasm
Urgent surgical referral	X-ray ± CT scan		CBC, ESR, ± CRP, MRI

Go to 'Primary conservative therapy 4–6 weeks'

No

Pertinent finding?

Yes

Fracture Surgical referral or conservative therapy as indicated	**Infection** Antibiotic ± surgical therapy	**Neoplasm** Definitive or palliative therapy

A. Primary (acute) conservative therapy
Education
Advice to stay active (avoid bedrest)
Heat
Acetaminophen
NSAIDs
Muscle relaxants
Tramadol
Opiates (consider very briefly for severe pain)
Manipulation

*Conservative therapy is recommended **only** if there are no signs of radiculopathy and includes severe radiculopathy with weakness among the red flags

B. Secondary (subacute/chronic) conservative therapy
Adjuvant neuropathic pain treatment, eg, TCAs, gabapentin or pregabalin
Exercise
Massage
Physical therapy
Pain management modalities
Acupuncture
Cognitive-behavioural therapy
Multidisiplinary rehabilitation program

Red flags for low back pain and associated diagnoses of concern

	Cauda equina syndrome	Fracture	Malignancy	Infection
Age >70 years		X	X	
Minor trauma with age >50 years		X	X	
Significant trauma		X		
Unexplained fever				X
Recent urinary infection; skin infection or penetrating wound near spine				X
Unrelenting night or rest pain			X	X
Progressive or disabling neurologic deficit (saddle anaesthesia, bilateral sciatica, bilateral leg weakness, difficulty voiding, faecal incontinence)	X		X	
Unexplained weight loss			X	
History or strong suspicion of cancer			X	
Osteoporosis		X		
Chronic steroid use		X		X
Immunosuppression				X
Intravenous drug abuse				X
Lack of improvement after 6 weeks of conservative therapy			X	X

Table 8.4 Red flags for low back pain and associated diagnoses of concern. Adapted from Kinkade [80] and Davis et al [81].

between those given IM steroids and those given placebo. Secondary outcomes were also comparable between the treatment groups. No serious adverse events were observed [78].

Treatment algorithm

Many pharmacological options for the treatment of radicular pain have been outlined in this chapter. Other pharmacological agents as well as nonpharmacological therapies may also be used, depending on the length and degree of pain. Figure 8.6 and Table 8.4 outlines a suggested treatment algorithm [79–81].

References

1   Mens JMA, Chavannes AW, Koes BW, et al. NHG-Standaard Lumbosacraal radiculair syndroom (in Dutch). *Huisarts Wet.* 2005;48:171-178.
2   Koes BW, van Tulder MW, Peul WC. Diagnosis and treatment of sciatica. *BMJ.* 2007;334:1313-1317.
3   Chou R, Qaseem A, Snow V, et al. Diagnosis and treatment of low back pain: a joint clinical practice guideline from the American College of Physicians and the American Pain Society. *Ann Intern Med.* 2007;147:478-491.
4   Chou R, Huffman LH. Medications for acute and chronic low back pain: a review of the evidence for an American Pain Society/American College of Physicians clinical practice guideline. *Ann Intern Med.* 2007;147:505-514.
5   North American Spine Society. Evidence-based clinical guidelines for multidisciplinary spine care. Available at: www.spine.org/Pages/PracticePolicy/ClinicalCare/ClinicalGuidelines/Default.aspx. Accessed September 25, 2012.
6   Boswell MV, Trescot AM, Datta S, et al. Interventional techniques: evidence-based practice guidelines in the management of chronic spinal pain. *Pain Physician.* 2007;10:7-111.
7   Hickey RF. Chronic low back pain: a comparison of diflunisal with paracetamol. *N Z Med J.* 1982;95:312-314.
8   Lee C, Straus WL, Balshaw R, Barlas S, Vogel S, Schnitzer TJ. A comparison of the efficacy and safety of nonsteroidal antiinflammatory agents versus acetaminophen in the treatment of osteoarthritis: a meta-analysis. *Arthritis Rheum.* 2004;51:746-754.
9   Towheed TE, Maxwell L, Judd MG, Catton M, Hochberg MC, Wells G. Acetaminophen for osteoarthritis. *Cochrane Database Syst Rev.* 2006;1:CD004257.
10 Wegman A, van der Windt D, van Tulder M, Stalman W, de Vries T. Nonsteroidal antiinflammatory drugs or acetaminophen for osteoarthritis of the hip or knee? A systematic review of evidence and guidelines. *J Rheumatol.* 2004;31:344-354.
11 Zhang W, Jones A, Doherty M. Does paracetamol (acetaminophen) reduce the pain of osteoarthritis? A meta-analysis of randomised controlled trials. *Ann Rheum Dis.* 2004;63:901-907.
12 Dart RC, Green JL, Bogdan GM. The safety profile of sustained release paracetamol during therapeutic use and following overdose. *Drug Saf.* 2005;28:1045-1056.
13 Fontana RJ. Acute liver failure including acetaminophen overdose. *Med Clin North Am.* 2008;92:761-794.
14 Porter RW, Ralston SH. Pharmacological management of back pain syndromes. *Drugs.* 1994;48:189-198.
15 Vroomen PC, de Krom MC, Slofstra PD, Knottnerus JA. Conservative treatment of sciatica: a systematic review. *J Spinal Disord.* 2000;13:463-469.
16 Roelofs PD, Deyo RA, Koes BW, Scholten RJ, van Tulder MW. Non-steroidal anti-inflammatory drugs for low back pain. *Cochrane Database Syst Rev.* 2008;1:CD000396.
17 Valat JP, Genevay S, Marty M, Rozenberg S, Koes B. Sciatica. *Best Pract Res Clin Rheumatol.* 2010;24:241-252.
18 Roelofs PDDM, Deyo RA, Koes BW, Scholten RJPM, van Tulder MW. Non-steroidal anti-inflammatory drugs for low back pain. *Cochrane Database Syst Rev.* 2008;1:CD000396.
19 Ong CK, Lirk P, Tan CH, Seymour RA. An evidence-based update on nonsteroidal anti-inflammatory drugs. *Clin Med Res.* 2007;5:19-34.
20 Moore RA, Derry S, Makinson GT, McQuay HJ. Tolerability and adverse events in clinical trials of celecoxib in osteoarthritis and rheumatoid arthritis: systematic review and meta-analysis of information from company clinical trial reports. *Arthritis Res Ther.* 2005;7:R644-R665.
21 Kearney PM, Baigent C, Godwin J, Halls H, Emberson JR, Patrono C. Do selective cyclo-oxygenase-2 inhibitors and traditional non-steroidal anti-inflammatory drugs increase the risk of atherothrombosis? Meta-analysis of randomised trials. *BMJ.* 2006;332:1302-1308.

22 Morlion B. Pharmacotherapy of low back pain: targeting nociceptive and neuropathic pain components. *Curr Med Res Opin*. 2011;27:11-33.

23 Attal N, Perrot S, Fermanian J, Bouhassira D. The neuropathic components of chronic low back pain: a prospective multicenter study using the DN4 questionnaire. *J Pain*. 2011;12:1080-1087.

24 Forde G. Adjuvant analgesics for the treatment of neuropathic pain: evaluating efficacy and safety profiles. *J Pract Manage*. 2007;56(suppl 2):3-12.

25 Fakata KL, Lipman AG. Pharmacotherapy for pain in rheumatologic conditions: the neuropathic component. *Curr Pain Headache Rep*. 2003;7:197-205.

26 Gore M, Dukes E, Rowbotham DJ, Tai K-S, Leslie D. Clinical characteristics and pain management among patients with painful peripheral neuropathic disorders in general practice settings. *Eur J Pain*. 2007;11:652-664.

27 O'Connor AB, Dworkin RH. Treatment of neuropathic pain: an overview of recent guidelines. *Am J Med*. 2009;122(10 suppl):S22-S32.

28 Fanciullo GJ, Ball PA, Girault G, Rose RJ, Hanscom B, Weinstein KJ. An observational study on the prevalence and pattern of opioid use in 25,479 patients with spine and radicular pain. *Spine*. 2002;27:201-205.

29 Hale ME, Fleischmann R, Salzman R, et al. Efficacy and safety of controlled-release versus immediate-release oxycodone: randomized, double-blind evaluation in patients with chronic back pain. *Clin J Pain*. 1999;15:179-183.

30 Hale ME, Dvergsten C, Gimbel J. Efficacy and safety of oxymorphone extended release in chronic low back pain: results of a randomized, double-blind, placebo- and active-controlled phase III study. *J Pain*. 2005;6:21-28.

31 Deyo RA, Smith DHM, Johnson ES, et al. Opioids for back pain patients: primary care prescribing patterns and use of services. *J Am Board Fam Med*. 2011;24:717-727.

32 Tzschentke TM, Christoph T, Kögel B, et al. (1R,2R)-3-(3-dimethylamino-1-ethyl-2-methyl-propyl)-phenol hydrochloride (tapentadol HCl): a novel μ-opioid receptor agonist/norepinephrine reuptake inhibitor with broad-spectrum analgesic properties. *J Pharmacol Exp Ther*. 2007;323:265-276.

33 Hale M, Upmalis D, Okamoto A, Lange C, Rauschkolb C. Tolerability of tapentadol immediate release in patients with lower back pain or osteoarthritis of the hip or knee over 90 days: a randomized, double-blind study. *Curr Med Res Opin*. 2009;25:1095-1104.

34 Hartrick C, van Hove I, Stegmann, J-U, et al. Advances in perioperative pain management: use of medications with dual analgesic mechanisms, tramadol and tapentadol. *Anesthesiology Clinics*. 2010;28:647-666.

35 Sullivan M. Opioid therapy for chronic pain: promise and peril. In: Proceedings from the 14th World Congress on Pain, Milan, Italy; August 27-31, 2012.

36 Staiger TO, Gaster B, Sullivan MD, Deyo RA. Systematic review of antidepressants in the treatment of chronic low back pain. *Spine*. 2003;28:2540-2545.

37 Atkinson JH, Slater MA, Williams RA, et al. A placebo-controlled randomized clinical trial of nortriptyline for chronic low back pain. *Pain*. 1998;76:287-296.

38 Khoromi S, Cui L, Nackers L, Max MB. Morphine, nortriptyline and their combination vs. placebo in patients with chronic lumbar root pain. *Pain*. 2007;130:66-75.

39 Williams JW Jr, Mulrow CD, Chiquette E, Noël PH, Aguilar C, Cornell J. A systematic review of new pharmacotherapies for depression in adults: evidence report summary. *Ann Intern Med*. 2000;132:743-756.

40 Cheng JK, Chiou LC. Mechanisms of the antinociceptive action of gabapentin. *J Pharmacol Sci*. 2006;100:471-486.

41 Attal N, Cruccu G, Baron R, et al. EFNS guidelines on the pharmacological treatment of neuropathic pain: 2010 revision. *Eur J Neurol*. 2010;17:1113-e88.

42 Moore RA, Wiffen PJ, Derry S, McQuay HJ. Gabapentin for chronic neuropathic pain and fibromyalgia in adults. *Cochrane Database Syst Rev*. 2011;3:CD007938.

43 Yildirim K, Sisecioglu M, Karatay S, et al. The effectiveness of gabapentin in patients with chronic radiculopathy. *Pain Clinic*. 2003;15:213-218.

44 Yildirim K, Deniz O, Gureser G, et al. Gabapentin monotherapy in patients with chronic radiculopathy: the efficacy and impact on life quality. *J Back Musculoskelet Rehab.* 2009;22:17-20.

45 Kasimcan O, Kaptan H. Efficacy of gabapentin for radiculopathy caused by lumbar spinal stenosis and lumbar disk hernia. *Neurol Med Chir.* 2010;50:1070-1073.

46 Gajraj NM. Pregabalin: its pharmacology and use in pain management. *Anesth Analg.* 2007;105:1805-1815.

47 Jones DL, Sorkin LS. Systemic gabapentin and S(+)-3-isobutyl-γ-aminobutyric acid block secondary hyperalgesia. *Brain Res.* 1998;810:93-99.

48 Bockbrader HN, Wesche D, Miller R, Chapel S, Janiczek N, Burger P. A comparison of the pharmacokinetics and pharmacodynamics of pregabalin and gabapentin. *Clin Pharmacokinet.* 2010;49:661-669.

49 Su TZ, Feng MR, Weber ML. Mediation of highly concentrative uptake of pregabalin by L-type amino acid transport in Chinese hamster ovary and Caco-2 cells. *J Pharmacol Exp Ther.* 2005;313:1406-1415.

50 Saldaña MT, Navarro A, Pérez C, Masramón X, Rejas J. Patient-reported-outcomes in subjects with painful lumbar or cervical radiculopathy treated with pregabalin: evidence from medical practice in primary care settings. *Rheumatol Int.* 2010;30:1005-1015.

51 Saldaña MT, Navarro A, Pérez C, Masramón X, Rejas J. A cost-consequences analysis of the effect of pregabalin in the treatment of painful radiculopathy under medical practice conditions in primary care settings. *Pain Pract.* 2010;10:31-41.

52 Baron R, Freynhagen R, Tölle TR, et al. The efficacy and safety of pregabalin in the treatment of neuropathic pain associated with chronic lumbosacral radiculopathy. *Pain.* 2010;150:420-427.

53 Toelle TR, Varvara R, Nimour M, Emir B, Brasser M. Pregabalin in neuropathic pain related to DPN, cancer and back pain: analysis of a 6-week observational study. *Open Pain J.* 2012;5:1-11.

54 Romanò CL, Romanò D, Bonora C, Mineo G. Pregabalin, celecoxib, and their combination for treatment of chronic low back pain. *J Orthopaed Traumatol.* 2009;10:185-191.

55 Semel D, Murphy TK, Zlateva G, Cheung R, Emir B. Evaluation of the safety and efficacy of pregabalin in older patients with neuropathic pain: results from a pooled analysis of 11 clinical studies. *BMC Fam Pract.* 2010;11:85.

56 North American Spine Society. Evidence-based clinical guidelines for multidisciplinary spine care. Diagnosis and treatment of degenerative lumbar spinal stenosis. Available at: www.spine.org/Pages/PracticePolicy/ClinicalCare/ClinicalGuidlines/Default.aspx. Accessed September 25, 2012.

57 Luijsterburg PA, Verhagen AP, Ostelo RW, van Os TA, Peul WC, Koes BW. Effectiveness of conservative treatments for the lumbosacral radicular syndrome: a systematic review. *Eur Spine J.* 2007;16:881-899.

58 Genevay S, Atlas SJ. Lumbar spinal stenosis. *Best Pract Res Clin Rheumatol.* 2010;24:253-265.

59 Parr AT, Diwan S, Abdi S. Lumbar interlaminar epidural injections in managing chronic low back and lower extremity pain: a systematic review. *Pain Physician.* 2009;12:163-188.

60 Conn A, Buenaventura RM, Datta S, Abdi S, Diwan S. Systematic review of caudal epidural injections in the management of chronic low back pain. *Pain Physician.* 2009;12:109-135.

61 Stout A. Epidural steroid injections for cervical radiculopathy. *Phys Med Rehabil Clin N Am.* 2011;22:149-159.

62 Carragee EJ, Hurwitz EL, Cheng I, et al. Treatment of neck pain: injections and surgical interventions: results of the Bone and Joint Decade 2000-2010 Task Force on Neck Pain and Its Associated Disorders. *Spine.* 2008;33:S153-S169.

63 Kwon JW, Lee JW, Kim SH, et al. Cervical interlaminar epidural steroid injection for neck pain and cervical radiculopathy: effect and prognostic factors. *Skeletal Radiol.* 2007;36:431-436.

64 Lee SH, Kim KT, Kim DH, Lee BJ, Son ES, Kwack YH. Clinical outcomes of cervical radiculopathy following epidural steroid injection: a prospective study with follow-up for more than 2 years. *Spine.* 2011;37:1041-1047.

65 Dawkins CJM. An analysis of the complications of extradural and caudal blocks. *Anaesthesia.* 1969;24:554–563.

66 Johnson A, Ryan MD, Roche J. Depo-medrol and myelographic arachnoiditis. *Med J Aust.* 1991;155:18–20.

67 Price C, Arden N, Coglan L, Rogers P. Cost-effectiveness and safety of epidural steroids in the management of sciatica. *Health Technol Assess.* 2005;9:1-58.

68 Abram SE, O'Connor TC. Complications associated with epidural steroid injections. *Reg Anesth.* 1996;21:149-162.

69 McGrath JM, Schaefer MP, Malkamaki DM. Incidence and characteristics of complications from epidural steroid injections. *Pain Med.* 2011;12:726-731.

70 Riew KD, Yin Y, Gilula L, et al. The effect of nerve-root injections on the need for operative treatment of lumbar radicular pain. A prospective, randomized, controlled, double-blind study. *J Bone Joint Surg Am.* 2000;82-A:1589-1593.

71 Karppinen J, Malmivaara A, Kurunlahti M, et al. Periradicular infiltration for sciatica: a randomized controlled trial. *Spine.* 2001;26:1059-1067.

72 Vad VB, Bhat AL, Lutz GE, Cammisa F. Transforaminal epidural steroid injections in lumbosacral radiculopathy: a prospective randomized study. *Spine.* 2002;27:11-16.

73 Thomas E, Cyteval C, Abiad L, Picot MC, Taourel P, Blotman F. Efficacy of transforaminal versus interspinous corticosteroid injection in discal radiculalgia - a prospective, randomised, double-blind study. *Clin Rheumatol.* 2003;22:299-304.

74 Schaufele MK, Hatch L, Jones W. Interlaminar versus transforaminal epidural injections for the treatment of symptomatic lumbar intervertebral disc herniations. *Pain Physician.* 2006;9:361-366.

75 Abdi S, Datta S, Trescot AM, et al. Epidural steroids in the management of chronic spinal pain: a systematic review. *Pain Physician.* 2007;10:185-212.

76 Scanlon GC, Moeller-Bertram T, Romanowsky SM, Wallace MS. Cervical transforaminal epidural steroid injections: more dangerous than we think? *Spine.* 2007;32:1249-1256.

77 Finckh A, Zufferey P, Schurch M-A, Balagué F, Waldburger M, So AKL. Short-term efficacy of intravenous pulse glucocorticoids in acute discogenic sciatica: a randomized controlled trial. *Spine.* 2006;31:377-381.

78 Friedman BW, Holden L, Esses D, et al. Parenteral corticosteroids for emergency department patients with non-radicular low back pain. *J Emerg Med.* 2006;31:365-370.

79 Duffy RL. low back pain: an approach to diagnosis and management. *Prim Care.* 2010;37:729-741.

80 Kinkade S. Evaluation and treatment of acute low back pain. *Am Fam Physician.* 2007;75:1181-8, 1190-1192.

81 Davis PC, Wippold FJ II, Cornelius RS, et al; for the American College of Radiology. ACR appropriateness criteria: low back pain. Available at: www.guideline.gov/content.aspx?id=35145. Accessed September 25, 2012.

Development of this book was supported by funding from Pfizer

Printed by Printforce, the Netherlands